THE ESSENTIALS OF PERITONEAL DIALYSIS

THE ESSENTIALS OF PERITONEAL DIALYSIS

Ramesh Khanna, MD
Health Sciences Center, University of Missouri, Columbia, Missouri, USA

Karl D. Nolph, MD
Health Sciences Center, University of Missouri, Columbia, Missouri, USA

and

Dimitrios G. Oreopoulos, MD PhD
Toronto Western Hospital, University of Toronto, Toronto, Canada

Illustrated by Bernard Tardieu

Springer-Science+Business Media, B.V.

Library of Congress Cataloging-in-Publication Data

```
Khanna, Ramesh.
   The essentials of peritoneal dialysis / Ramesh Khanna, Karl D.
 Nolph, and Dimitrios G. Oreopoulos.
       p.   cm.
   Includes bibliographical references and index.
   ISBN 978-94-010-5223-8        ISBN 978-94-011-2755-4 (eBook)
   DOI 10.1007/978-94-011-2755-4
   1. Peritoneal dialysis.   I. Nolph, Karl D.  II. Oreopoulos, D. G.
 (Dimitrios G.)  III. Title.
   [DNLM: 1. Peritoneal Dialysis.   WJ 378 K45e]
 RC901.7.P48K43  1992
 617.4'61059--dc20
 DNLM/DLC
 for Library of Congress                                92-17615
```

Printed on acid-free paper

TABLE OF CONTENTS

Preface   ix

1. Physiology of peritoneal dialysis   1
   The peritoneal cavity   4
   Normal peritoneum   4
   Uremic peritoneum   6
   The peritoneum in CAPD   6
      Blood supply   7
      Lymphatic drainage   8
      Solute and water transport across the peritoneum   9
      The kinetics of ultrafiltration during peritoneal dialysis   13
      Solute equilibration, ultrafiltration volumes, and peritoneal
         membrane transport characteristics   15
      Interpretation of peritoneal equilibration test results   18

2. Peritoneal access   19
   Bedside access for acute peritoneal dialysis   19
   Long-term peritoneal access   21
   Preinsertion patient preparation   22
   Peritoneoscopic technique   22
   Surgical technique   25
   Creation of a subcutaneaous tunnel   27
   Post-operative care   30
   Catheter break-in   31
   Subsequent catheter care   32
   Exit-site care   33
   Indications for catheter removal   33

3. **Techniques, prescriptions, and indications**   35
    Intermittent regimes   35
    Continuous regimes   37
    Alternate PD regimes   39

4. **Dialysis solutions and equipment**   45
    Dialysis solution   45
    Transfer sets   46
        Steps of a solution exchange with a straight transfer set   50
        The basic Y-set procedure   50
    Assist devices for CAPD   51
        Ultraviolet light devices   51
        Sterile connection device   51
    Peritoneal dialysis machines   53

5. **Acute peritoneal dialysis**   54
    Access for acute peritoneal dialysis   54
    Catheter complications   56
    Prescription of acute peritoneal dialysis   60

6. **Automated peritoneal dialysis**   64

7. **Adequacy of dialysis**   69
    Clinical indicators   69
    Adequacy indices   70
    Creatinine clearance measurements   70
    Urea kinetic parameters   73
    Mass transfer area coefficient   75

8. **Peritonitis and exit-site infection**   76
    Diagnosis of peritonitis   78
    Management of peritonitis   83
    Early treatment   83

9. **Complications during peritoneal dialysis**   89
    Uremic organ dysfunction during CAPD   89
        Nutritional problems   89
        Abnormalities of lipid metabolism   92
        Hematological problems   92
        Hypertension   93
        Renal osteodystrophy   93
        Neurological complications   94

Pericarditis   94
Vascular problems   95
Endocrine function   95
Acquired cystic disease of the kidney   96
Complications due to peritoneal dialysis   96
Pressure-related complications   96
Insufficient ultrafiltration   97

10. Peritoneal dialysis in diabetics   99
Why choose CAPD over other dialysis therapies?   99
What is the ideal time to initiate dialysis in diabetics?   100
Peritoneal access   100
Is glucose an ideal osmotic agent for diabetic CAPD patients?   101
Dialysis regimens and blood-sugar control   101
Intermittent peritoneal dialysis   101
Continuous cyclic peritoneal dialysis   102
Continuous ambulatory peritoneal dialysis   102
Blood-sugar control in CAPD patients   102
Intraperitoneal insulin   103
Short-term and long-term outcomes   105

11. Peristoneal dialysis in children   109
Peritoneal physiology   109
Peritoneal access   110
Acute renal failure   110
End-stage renal disease   111

Literature for further reading   113

Index   119

PREFACE

The goal of writing this book was to provide a simplified, yet up-to-date view of peritoneal dialysis and to deal concisely with all its aspects. To achieve this aim, the book is written in a style that even a beginner with very little knowledge of dialysis would be able to benefit from its contents. It is also intended as an overview of the fundamentals of peritoneal dialysis for medicine trainees. Moreover, it should also be helpful to those nephrologists who are lacking in experience with peritoneal dialysis. The text is succinct and emphasis is placed on illustrations and tables. Controversies are not explained in detail.

Familiarity with the contents of the book should help to establish a good foundation for those interested in eventually delving more deeply into the field of peritoneal dialysis. A comprehensive list of references for further reading is included at the end of the book. This book should be a valuable tool for those who desire only to become familiar with the fundamentals of the procedure using a readily understandable text.

The authors hope that this book meets not only the needs of internal medicine, nephrology, and nursing trainees, but also those who are, as yet, beginners to peritoneal dialysis.

Ramesh Khanna, MD
Karl D. Nolph, MD
Dimitrios G. Oreopoulos, MD, PhD

1 PHYSIOLOGY OF PERITONEAL DIALYSIS

Adequate peritoneal dialysis maintains an end-stage renal disease patient symptom-free by partially replacing some of the functions performed by the healthy kidneys.

Dialysis (a) removes solutes accumulated in the blood, such as urea nitrogen, creatinine, phosphate, potassium, water, etc., into the dialysis solution infused into the peritoneal cavity and (b) corrects acidosis by the addition of bicarbonate, by way of lactate, to the blood from the dialysis solution.

The dialysis takes place between the blood in the capillaries located in the interstitium of the peritoneum and the infused dialysis solution across the peritoneal membrane. The peritoneal membrane acts as an imperfect semipermeable membrane (allows small molecules and water to pass through faster than large molecules). The composition of the dialysis solution is near that of extra-cellular fluid. Tables 1–3 show fluid, electrolyte and acid-base balance, and adequacy of solute removal compared to a healthy kidney in a typical patient on continuous ambulatory peritoneal dialysis (CAPD).

TABLE 1. Comparison of water and electrolyte removal (on a liberal fluid and salt intake) between the healthy kidneys and CAPD

	Healthy kidneys	CAPD
Water removal (liter/day)	2	2
Sodium removal (mEq/day)	100–150	100–150
Potassium removal (mEq/day)	50	30 + fecal loss
Phosphate removal (mg/day)	800–1000	300

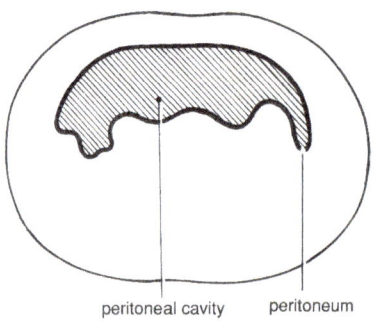

peritoneal cavity   peritoneum

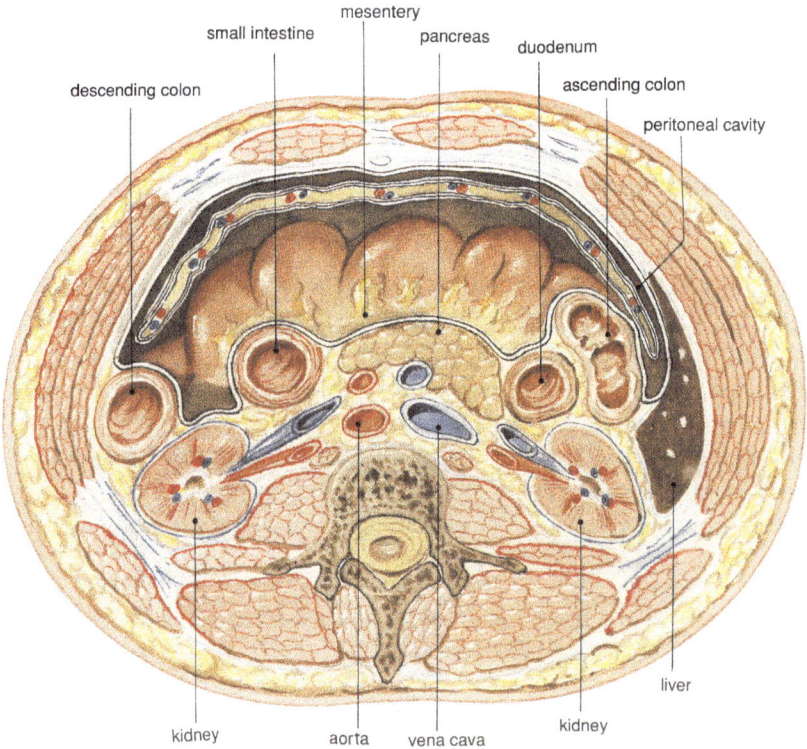

Figure 1A: Cross section showing the peritoneal cavity and the internal organs.

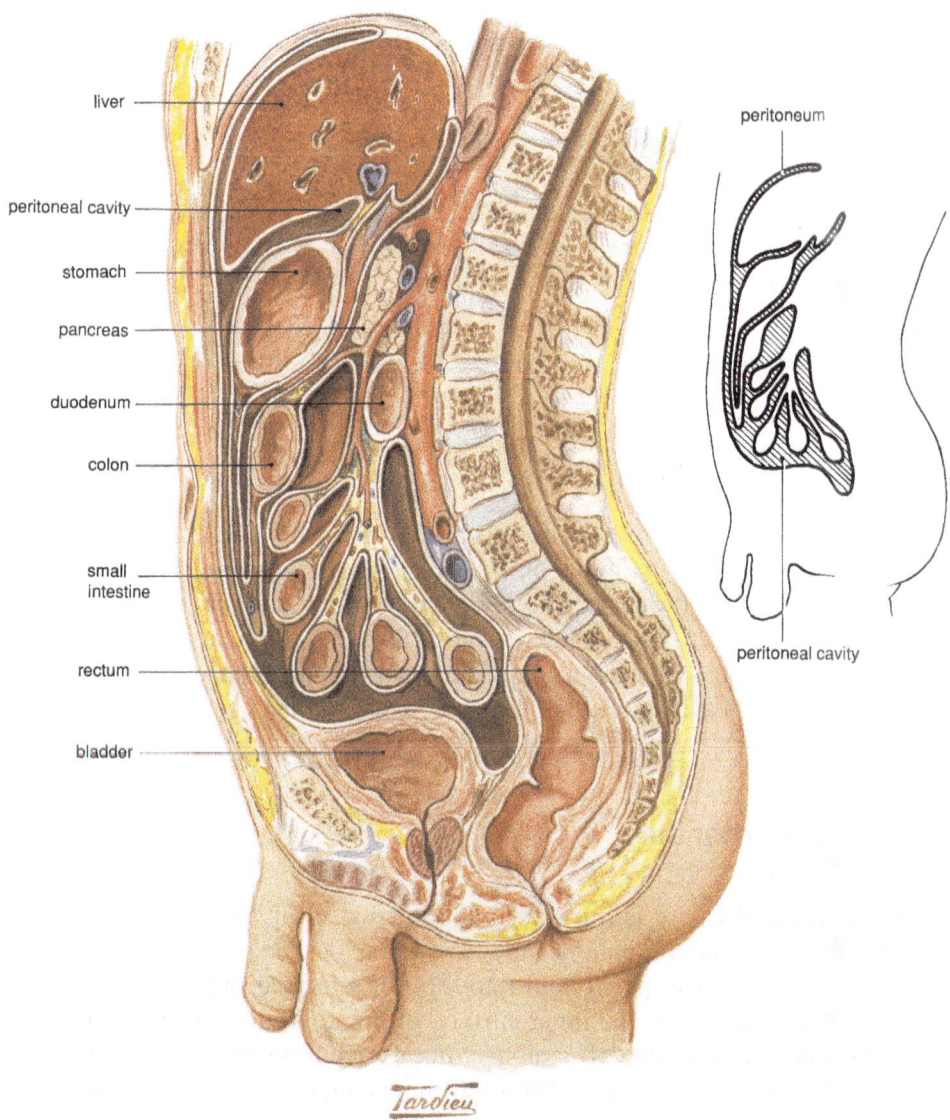

Figure 1B: Sagittal section showing the peritoneal cavity and the internal organs.

TABLE 2. Comparison of acid-base status between normal individuals and CAPD patients

	Normal individual	CAPD patient
pH	7.4	7.35–7.4
HCO_3 (mEq/liter)	24	22–24
PCO_2 (mmHg)	40	37–40

TABLE 3. Comparison of solute clearances/removal between healthy kidneys and CAPD

	Healthy kidneys	CAPD
Urea (liter/wk)	750	70
B12 (liter/wk)	1200	40
Inulin (liter/wk)	1200	30
$ß_2$ mcgb* (mg/wk)	1000	250

* $ß_2$ microglobulin.

The peritoneal cavity

The potential space between the partial and visceral peritoneum is called the peritoneal cavity (Figure 1). At any given time, under normal circumstances the peritoneal cavity contains a small amount (less than 10 ml) of fluid. This fluid contains phosphatidylcholine secreted by the mesothelial cells that lubricates the surface of the peritoneal membrane. The peritoneal cavity has the potential to accommodate large volumes of fluid as is seen in cases of chronic ascites.

Normal peritoneum

The peritoneal cavity is lined by a continuous serous membrane with a simple monolayered squamous mesothelium underlaid by connective tissue (Figure 2). The peritoneum covers the visceral organs (visceral peritoneum) and lines the inner surface of the abdominal wall (parietal peritoneum). Knowledge of peritoneal ultrastructure in normal and peritoneal dialysis patients comes from the independent extensive peritoneal biopsy studies by Dobby and Gotlieb. Mesothelial cells are flattened, elongated cells of 0.6 to 2 μ thickness. The luminal side of the mesothelial cells has numerous 2–3 μ long cytoplasmic extensions, the microvilli. They are believed to increase the peritoneal surface area up to 40 square meters. In addition, most cells bear a single cilium (Figure 2). Mesothelial cell boundaries are tortuous and adjacent cells often overlap. The peritoneal side of the intercellular space is closed by tight junctions and desmosomes. Mesothelial cell nuclei are oval or cigar shaped. Two prominent nucleoli are commonly observed. The cellular organelles consist of a prominent rough endoplasmic reticulum exhibiting ribosome-studded cisternae, a well developed Golgi apparatus, mitochondria, and 3–4 lipid inclusions with concentric whorls of electron dense lamellae. It is currently believed that these lipid inclusions represent packages of phospholipids which are synthesized in the cells and released by exocytotic extrusion onto the peritoneal surface. The submesothelial basement membrane is a thin, readily visible layer under the mesothelial cell layer. The interstitium is a layer of areolar tissue, 2–3 mm in thickness, composed of oriented bundles of collagen fibers set in a matrix of ground substances of moderate electron density. These collagen fibers form a mat of very fine reticular formation filling the interstitium. The fluid in the interstitium is entrapped in the

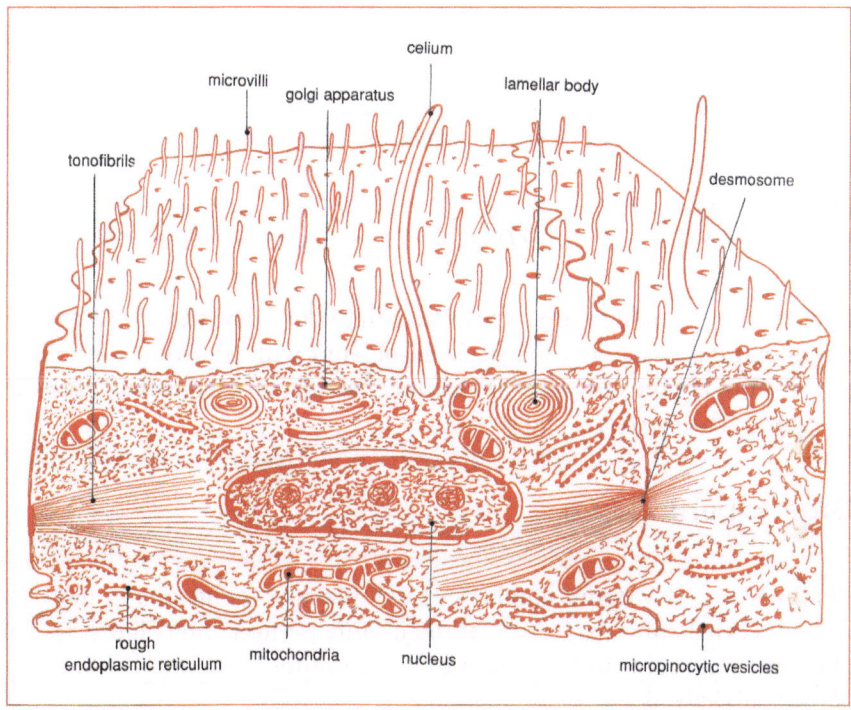

Figure 2: Diagramatic representation of a normal mesothelial cell. C: celium; P: micropinocytic vesicles; L: lamellar body; G: Golgi apparatus; M: mitochondria; D: desmosome; T: tonofibrils; RER rough endoplasmic reticulum; N: nucleus. (Adapted from Dobbi, Lloyd and Gall: Advances in Peritoneal Dialysis, Peritoneal Dialysis Bulletin, Inc., Toronto, 1990.)

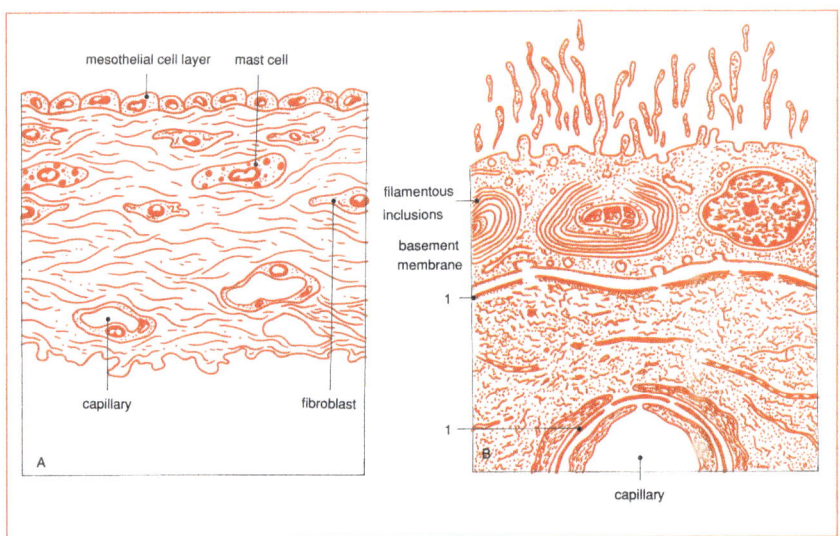

Figure 3: A: diagrammatic summary of morphological findings in peritoneal biopsies from uremic (non-dialyzed) patients. Light microscopic examination (LM) reveals no abnormality as compared to controls. B: Transmission electron microscopy (TEM) shows intracytoplasmic filamentous inclusions in mesothelial cells. Meso: mesothelial cell; MC: mast cell; Fb: fibroblast; CAP: capillary; BM: basement membrane. (Adapted from Dobbi, Lloyd and Gall: Advances in Peritoneal Dialysis, Peritoneal Dialysis Bulletin, Inc., Toronto, 1990.)

minute spaces among the proteoglycan filaments. The fluid flow through the interstitial tissue and matrix is associated with transport through the interstitium not only of water molecules, but also of electrolyte, nutrients, oxygen, carbon dioxide, and so forth.

Uremic peritoneum

The presence of varying numbers of cytoplasmic inclusions in mesothelial cells is a distinctive feature of the uremic peritoneum (Figure 3). This phenomenon seems to be a feature of the uremic state and is 'cured' by peritoneal dialysis.

The peritoneum in CAPD

Mesothelium subjected to the process of peritoneal dialysis undergoes reactive changes in response to the new environment (Figure 4). There appears to be a relative profileration of mesothelial cells giving an appearance of increased cells per unit area, and there is a diminution in the density of microvilli. Abnormal surface protuberances, such as blisters and blebs, are another altered feature of the peritoneum with dialysis. Hyperplasia of the rough endoplasmic reticulum is a characteristic feature of mesothelium in patients who have been treated with CAPD. Both diabetic and nondiabetic patients show reduplication of basement membranes of mesothelium and stromal blood vessels.

Blood supply

The superior mesenteric artery supplies the bulk of the visceral peritoneum and the underlying structures. The intercostal, epigastric, and lumbar arteries supply the parietal peritoneum. The venous blood of the visceral peritoneum is returned to the portal circulation, whereas the venous drainage of parietal peritoneum returns to the caval circulation. This is im-

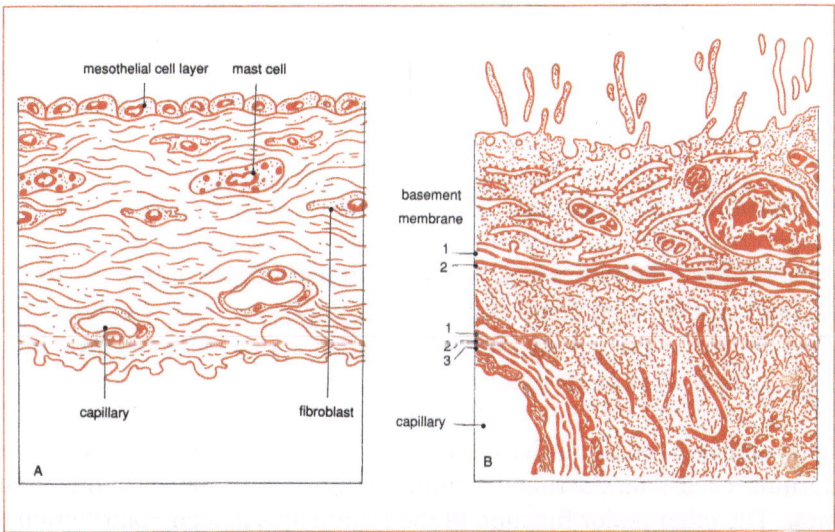

Figure 4: A: diagrammatic summary of morphological findings in peritoneal biopsies from CAPD patients. Light microscopic examinations (LM) may reveal no abnormality as compared to controls. B: Transmission electron microscopy (TEM) may show diminution in the density of microvilli and micropinocytotic vesicles but hyperplasia of the RER. Diabetic and non-diabetic patients may show reduplication of the basement membrane (BM: 1, 2, 3). Meso: mesothelial cell layer; MC: mast cell; Fb: fibroblast; RER: rough endoplasmic reticulum. (Adapted from Dobbi, Lloyd and Gall: Advances in Peritoneal Dialysis, Peritoneal Dialysis Bulletin, Inc., Toronto, Publishers 1990; 6:3.)

portant because drugs introduced intraperitoneally will be partly subjected to liver handling during their first circulatory pass. The capillaries of the parietal and visceral peritoneum exhibit a complex branching pattern.

Lymphatic drainage

Lymphatic drainage from the peritoneal cavity is mainly through specialized lymph stomata up to 22.5 μ in diameter located in the subdiaphragmatic peritoneum. The stomata are formed by the separation of adjacent mesothelial cells in the surrounding mesothelium. At the stomata, the mesothelial basement membrane and the underlying lattice of connective tissue become fenestrated and so allow the mesothelial cells and endothelial cells of the lymphatic capillaries to join together to form a channel from the peritoneal cavity to lymphatic lumen. The lymph vessels from the subdiaphragmatic area drain into collecting lymphatics within the muscular portion of the diaphragm. From the diaphragm and the diaphragmatic lymph nodes, most of the lymphatic trunks accompany the internal mammary vessels to the anterior mediastinal lymph nodes and thereafter return almost 80% of the lymphatic drainage to the venous circulation via the right lymph duct (Figure 5). Both in the parietal and visceral peritoneal interstitium a rich network of lymphatic vessels is observed. They drain mainly into the thoracic lymph duct.

Inspiratory and expiratory diaphragmatic movements appear to open and close the stomata which provide access to lymphatic lumen from the peritoneal cavity. Lymphatic contractility and the intrathoracic negative pressure aided by the presence of valves in the lumen of the lymph capillaries maintains the forward flow in the lymphatic vessels (Figure 6).

The lymphatics draining the peritoneal cavity act as a one-way system returning excess intraperitoneal fluid and protein to the systemic circulation. The other major function of the lymphatics is their contribution to the host defenses of the peritoneum by removing any foreign body that might enter the peritoneal cavity. The lymphatics draining the peritoneal cavity are the only pathway for absorption of intraperitoneal biologically inert particles, colloids, and cells. Several physiological factors such as respiratory rate, intraperitoneal hydrostatic pressure, body posture, and peritonitis influence the lymphatic flow rate. Although the lymphatics carrying fluids and solutes from the intestinal mucosa traverse the mesentery before draining into the thoracic duct, their contribution to absorption of fluid from the peritoneal cavity is unknown.

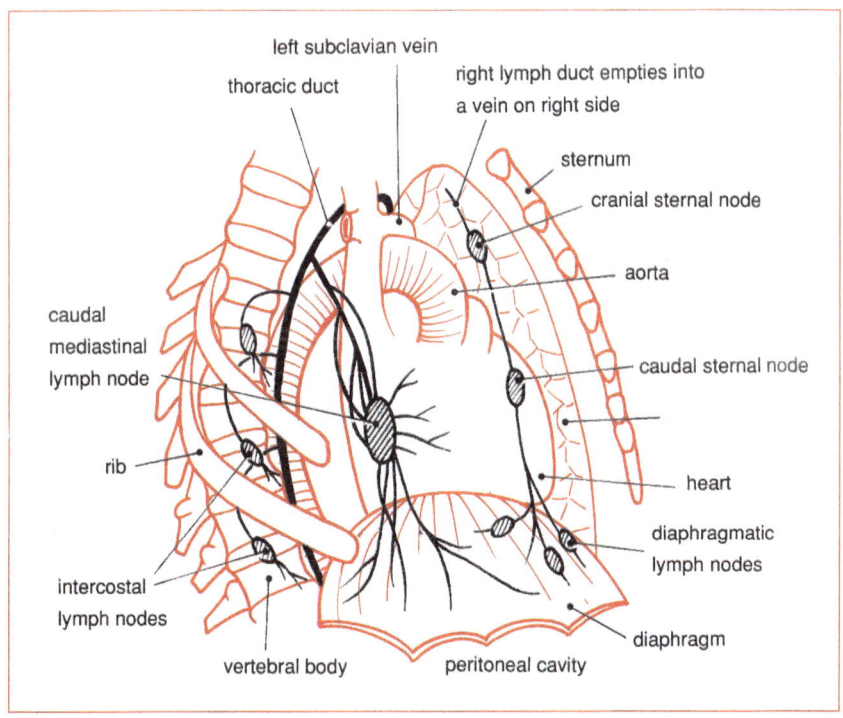

Figure 5: Lateral view of the thorax depicting the lymph drainage from the peritoneal cavity in sheep. (Modified from Abernethy et al., Am J Physiol 260: F353 1991.)

Solute and water transport across the peritoneum

Solute and water exchange between the peritoneal microcirculation and peritoneal cavity occurs across the peritoneal membrane by diffusion and convection. Ions diffuse in the same manner as whole molecules; colloid particles diffuse in a similar manner, except that because of their large size, they diffuse far less rapidly than small molecular substances. The peritoneal membrane behaves as an imperfect semipermeable membrane, i.e. permeable to water and substances of smaller size, and less permeable to large molecules. Substances such as water, and many of the dissolved ions, appear to pass through peritoneal membrane pores and intercellular clefts. Although the exact nature of these pores is unknown, substances with sizes considerably smaller than the pores readily pass through the peritoneum (Figure 7).

Diffusion is a spontaneous process whereby molecules or other particles in liquids reach uniform concentration via random movement throughout the solvent.

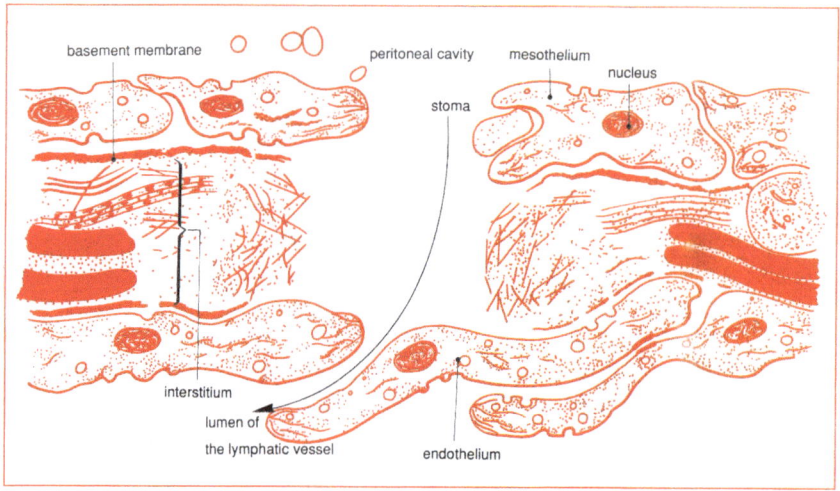

Figure 6: Schematic representation of a subdiaphragmatic stoma. (Adapted from Tsillibary and Wissig: Am J Anat 1987; 180:195.)

The net diffusion rate of a substance between the capillary and peritoneal cavity correlates positively with the solute concentration difference, the pressure difference across the membrane, the membrane area, and the temperature of the media; diffusion rate correlates negatively with the square root of the solute molecular weight and the thickness of the peritoneal membrane.

The process of net movement of water caused by a water concentration difference (osmotic pressure) is called osmotic ultrafiltration.

Bulk or convective flow is a transport mechanism for water and solutes during peritoneal dialysis exchanges. Because of either hydrostatic or osmotic pressure gradients across a membrane, during bulk flow, solutes and water move along this gradient at a rate often many times that which can be accounted for by net diffusion.

During bulk or convective flow, large numbers of molecules are moving in the same direction, streaming through the pores as part of the total fluid, as opposed to random movement in pure diffusion.

A substance with a molecular weight too great for it to move readily through the pores of a membrane, creates osmotic pressure across the

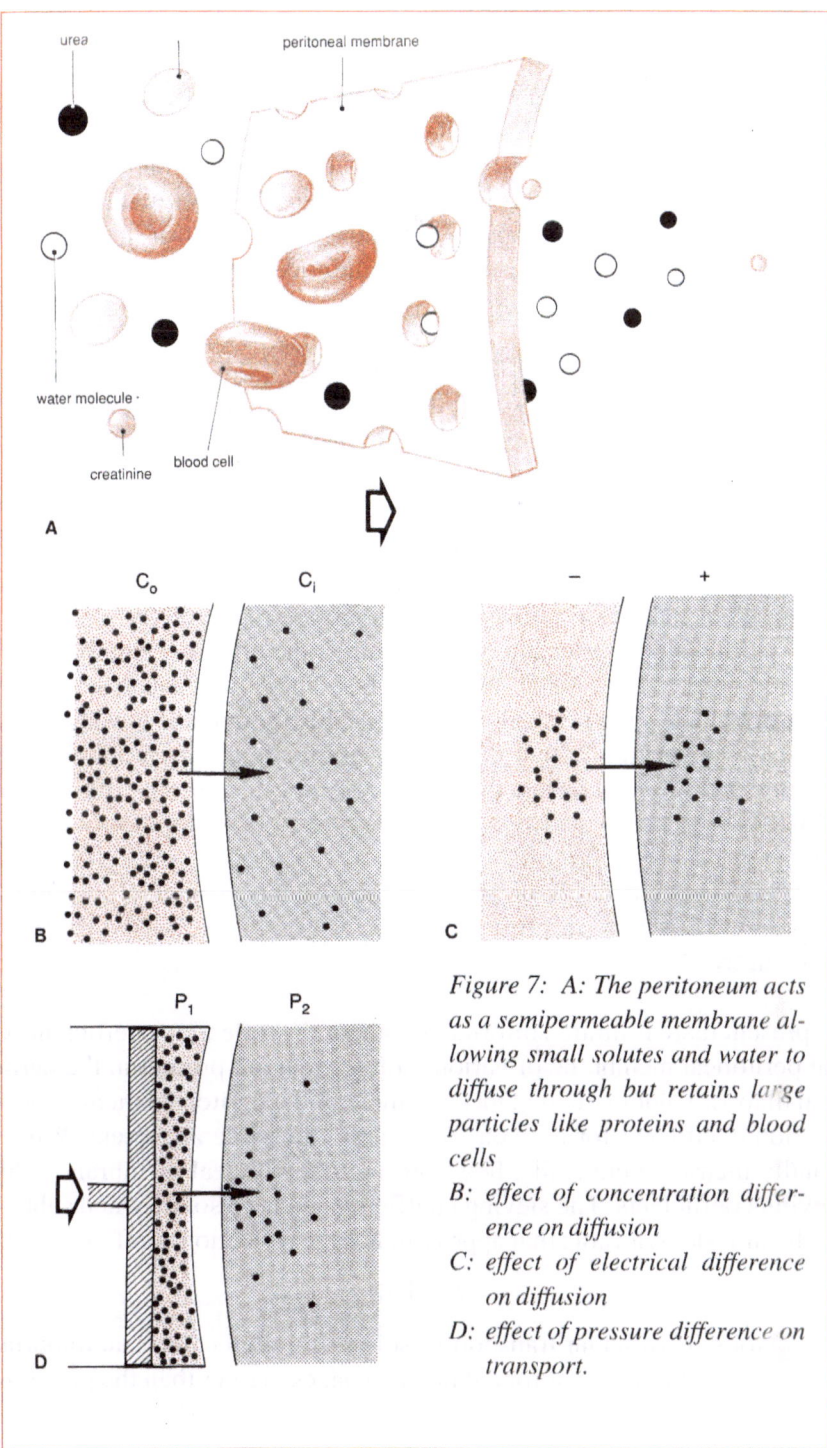

Figure 7: A: *The peritoneum acts as a semipermeable membrane allowing small solutes and water to diffuse through but retains large particles like proteins and blood cells*

B: *effect of concentration difference on diffusion*

C: *effect of electrical difference on diffusion*

D: *effect of pressure difference on transport.*

membrane. This pressure then acts in the same way as hydrostatic pressure does, causing bulk flow of water through the pores of the membrane. During convective flow, net removal of solutes such as sodium and potassium per liter of ultrafiltrate, is usually far below their respective concentrations in the extracellular fluid, indicating a sieving effect. The possible explanation for such electrolyte sieving is believed to be either a membrane feature or an interaction between molecules within membrane channels. Charged substances on all surfaces (Figure 7c) in the endothelial and mesothelial inter-cellular gaps on basement membranes or in the interstitial gel matrix, may play a role in impeding electrolyte movements with ultrafiltration.

> The sieving coefficient for any solute is the ratio of the concentration in the ultrafiltrate to that in the plasma water. It can have a maximum value of 1.0 (no membrane sieving) and a minimum value of 0.0 (total sieving).

The ability of a water soluble solute to exert an effective osmotic pressure gradient is a function of its molecular radius relative to the radius of the water-filled membrane pores. If the membrane is perfectly semipermeable (permeable to water but not to solutes), the effective and theoretical osmotic pressures are equal. However, for a membrane (such as the peritoneum) which is not perfectly semipermeable (permeable to water and to solutes to a varying extent depending upon solute size), the effective osmotic pressure will be less than the theoretic value because of the solute transfer.

> The effective osmotic pressure divided by the theoretical osmotic pressure has been defined by Staverman as the reflection coefficient (σ).

At present there is limited information about the reflection coefficients for the peritoneal membrane of various solutes that are present in the peritoneal dialysis solution. Direct measurement of the peritoneal membrane reflection coefficient for a given solute is not possible at present. What is usually measured clinically, however, is the peritoneal membrane solute sieving coefficients. The sieving coefficient (S) for a solute when subtracted from 1 yields a value that approximates the reflection coefficient (σ):

$$\sigma = 1 - S.$$

Pinocytotic or vesicular transport of solutes through cells is an important mechanism of movement for solutes with sizes greater than the pore sizes and macromolecules such as proteins. Small amounts of plasma proteins do leak through the pores in the capillary walls and may be transported through endothelium by pinocytosis into the interstitial spaces. Transport from there across the mesothelium into the peritoneal cavity may also be by pinocytosis. However, there is no evidence as yet to indicate that the reverse process occurs, i.e. macromolecules are returned to the blood across the capillary wall. The route for macromolecule absorption from the interstitium and peritoneal cavity is probably mainly through the lymphatics.

The kinetics of ultrafiltration during peritoneal dialysis

During peritoneal dialysis, glucose is used as an osmotic agent to induce ultrafiltration. Because of its reflection coefficient, glucose generates a high osmotic pressure which induces ultrafiltration from the blood. When two liters of dialysis solution containing glucose are introduced into the peritoneal cavity during peritoneal dialysis, the forces that are normally operative across the capillary are modified in favor of enhanced ultrafiltration. The net transcapillary ultrafiltration rate is maximal at the beginning of the exchange, when the glucose concentration gradient is maximum, and decreases exponentially as the glucose concentration gradient

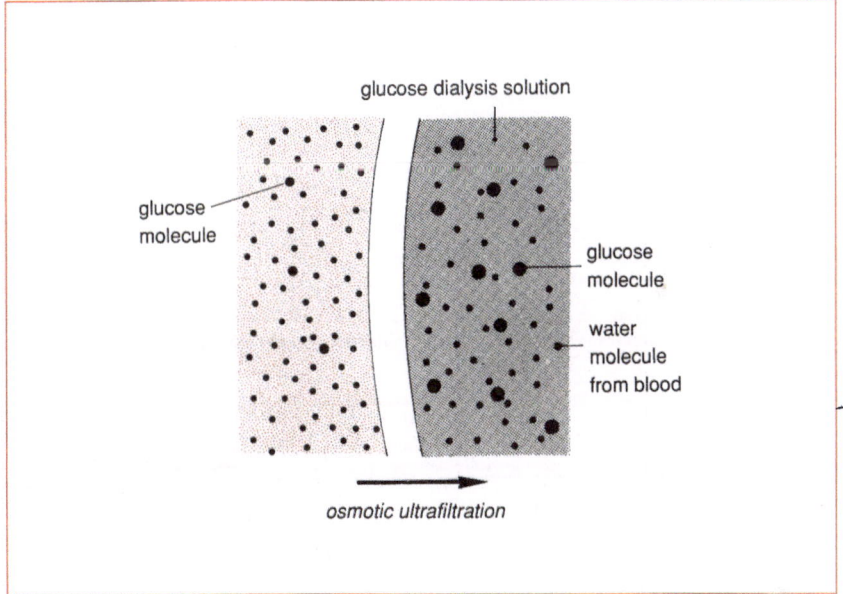

Figure 8: Osmotic ultrafiltration across the peritoneal membrane with a glucose dialysis solution in the peritoneal cavity.

is dissipated by a combination of glucose absorption and dilution by the ultrafiltrate (Figure 9).

Studies done in CAPD patients have shown that 2 liters of hypertonic (2.5% dextrose solution) dialysis solution, when infused and allowed to dwell for 4 hours in the peritoneal cavity, causes about 600 ml of cumulative ultrafiltration (Figure 10). During the same period, cumulative reabsorption of fluid from the peritoneal cavity would be about 200 ml. Thus, the net measurable ultrafiltration would be appreciably reduced to 400 ml. Peak intraperitoneal volume would be observed at about 2–3 hours after the dwell, when the reabsorption rate equals the ultrafiltration rate.

> The net transcapillary ultrafiltration rate is maximum at the beginning of an exchange, and ultrafiltration volume peaks at about 2–3 hours when transcapillary ultrafiltration equals reabsorption; intraperitoneal volume begins to decrease thereafter, probably because of continued lymph absorption.

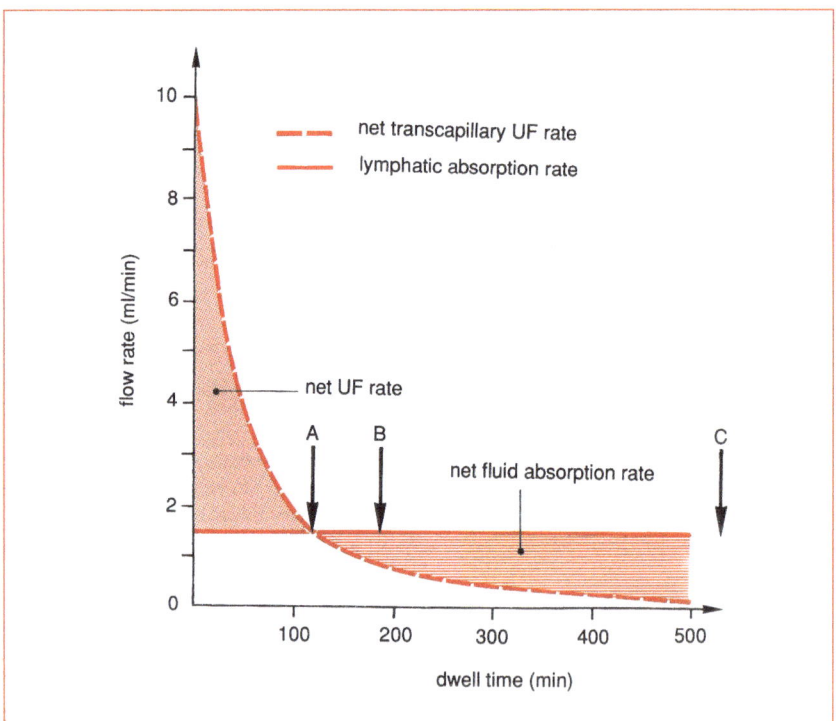

Figure 9: Kinetics of ultrafiltration during peritoneal dialysis. Arrow A: time of peak ultrafiltration; B: osmolar equilibrium; C: hypothetical glucose equilibrium.

From then on, the intraperitoneal volume begins to decrease, because the constant convective absorption rate exceeds the transcapillary ultrafiltration rate which, in turn, tends to decline because of a gradual dissipation of the glucose osmotic gradient. Glucose equilibrium is achieved much later, maybe as late as 6 to 10 hours after the infusion.

Solute equilibration, ultrafiltration volumes, and peritoneal membrane transport characteristics

Systematic measurements of peritoneal equilibration rates of urea, creatinine, glucose, protein, potassium, sodium, and drain and residual volumes in over 130 CAPD patients have yielded equilibration curves for these solutes during a 4 hour peritoneal dialysis exchange using 2.5% dextrose solution (Figure 11). The steps of the standardized peritoneal equilibration test are given in Table 4. Based on such peritoneal equilibration test results, the peritoneal equilibration rate can be categorized as low, low average, high average, and high (Figures 11A and B).

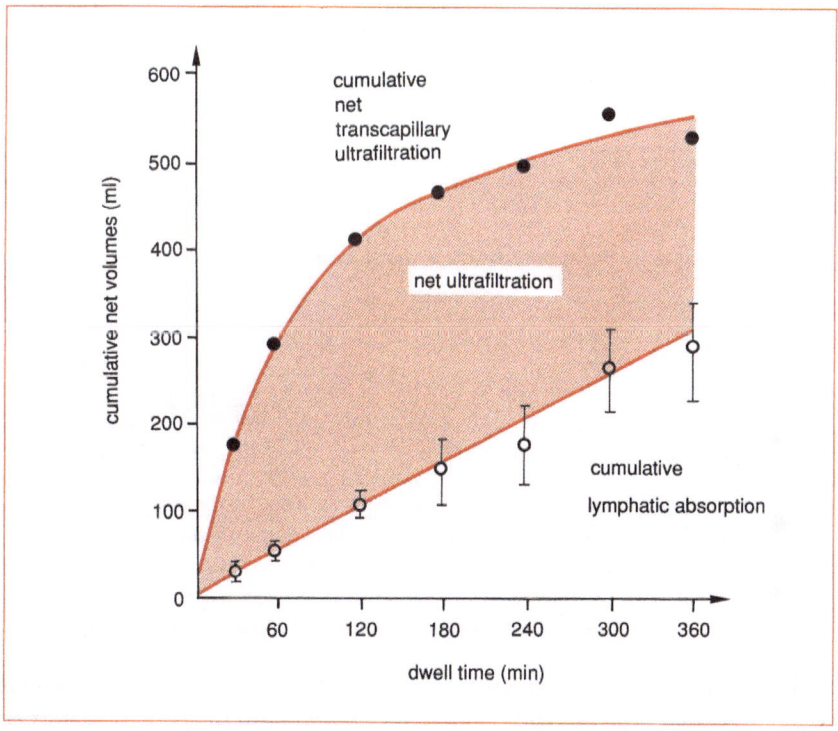

Figure 10: Cumulative transcapillary ultrafiltration, lymphatic absorption, and net ultrafiltration during hypertonic dextrose peritoneal dialysis exchanges in humans.

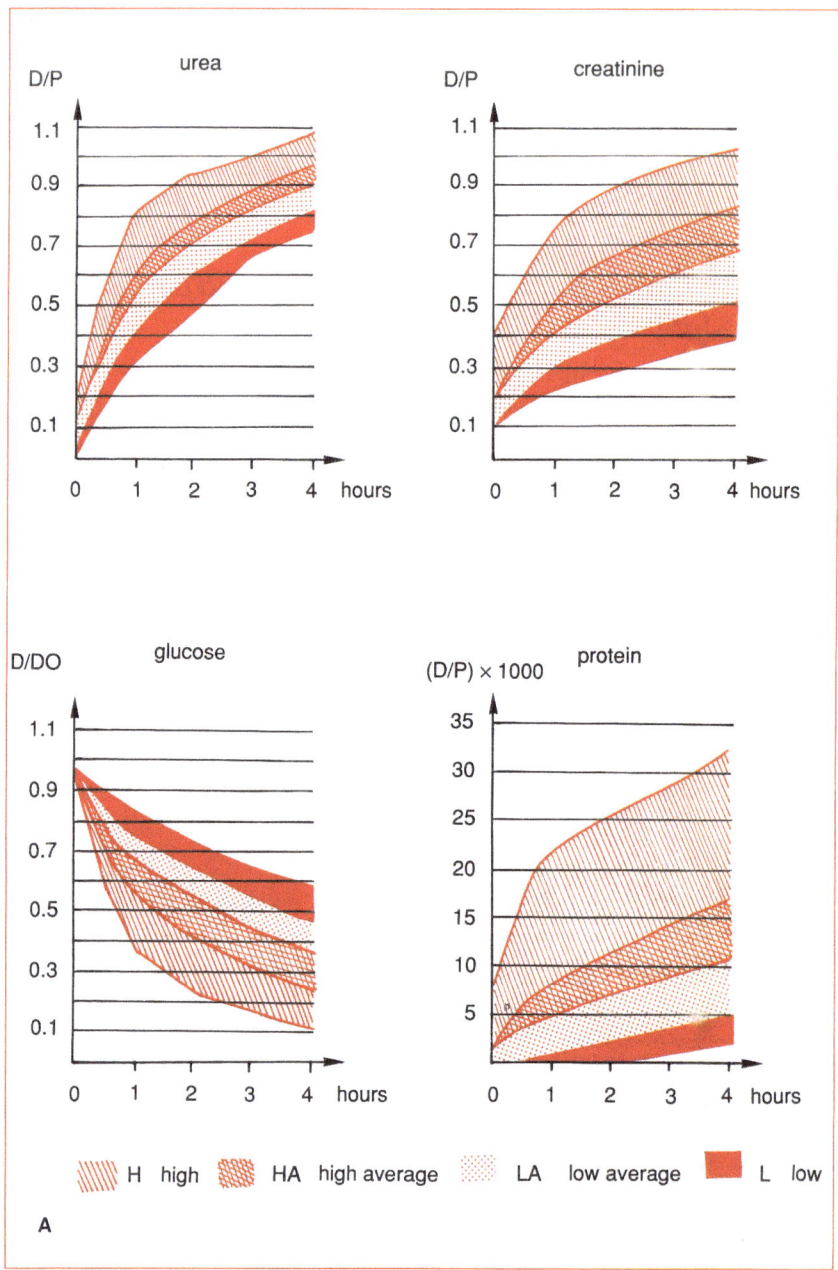

Figure 11A: The equilibration test results in a study population for urea, creatinine, glucose, and protein. Area shaded in different patterns portray results representing high (H), high average (HA), low average (LA), and low (L) peritoneal equilibration rates.
(Adapted from Twardowski et al., Peritoneal Dialysis Bulletin 7:138, 1987.)

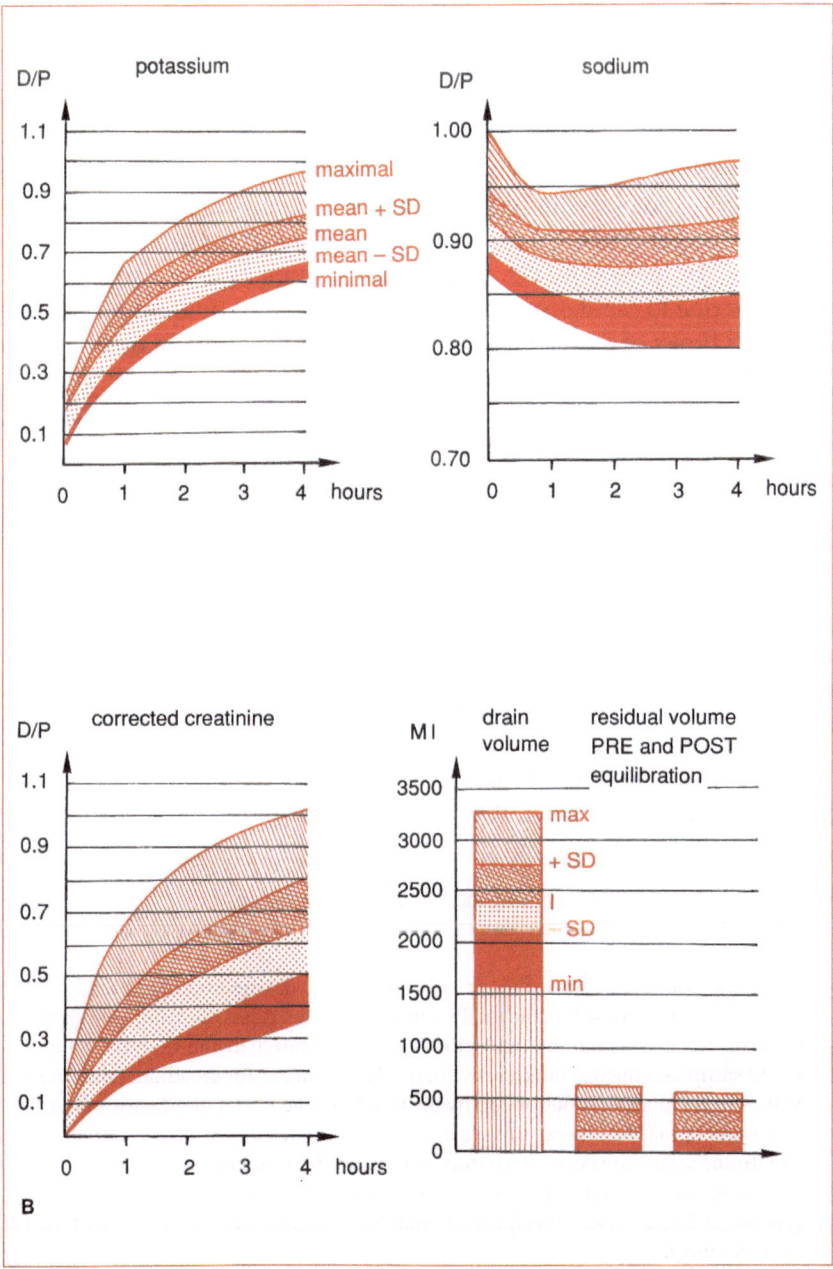

Figure 11B: The equilibration test results in a study population for potassium, sodium, corrected creatinine, with drain and residual volumes. Area shaded in different patterns portray results representing high (H), high average (HA), low average (LA), and low (L) peritoneal equilibration rates.
(Adapted from Twardowski et al., Peritoneal Dialysis Bulletin 7:138, 1987.)

Interpretation of peritoneal equilibration test results

In patients with low equilibration rates, peak ultrafiltration occurs late in an exchange. Ultrafiltration continues over many hours of dwell. Also, the dialysate to plasma ratios of various solutes increase almost lineary during an exchange; consequently, their clearances per exchange also increase almost linearly throughout the long exchange. Patients with high peritoneal equilibration rates have lower ultrafiltration during a 4 hour exchange. In these patients, peak ultrafiltration occurs early during an exchange due to rapid glucose absorption followed by fluid reabsorption. Beyond 4 hours of dwell, these patients will have minimal or no net ultrafiltration. Dialysate to plasma ratios of small solutes are close to unity by 4 hours. Also, the clearances of small solutes in long-dwell exchanges decreases proportionally due to the reduction of drain volume. Patients with solute equilibration rates between these two extremes have intermediate patterns.

TABLE 4.   The steps of the standardized peritoneal equilibration test

1. Patient performs an overnight exchange which should dwell for 8–12 hours.
2. Pretest exchange fluid is drained completely over 20 minutes in the sitting position.
3. 2 liters of 2.5% dialysis solution is infused at a rate of 200 ml/min. The patient should be in a supine position during infusion and, for better solution mixing, rolls over from side to side after each 400 ml infusion.
4. At the completion of infusion (0 dwell time), 200 ml of dialysis solution is drained into the bag, mixed well, a 10 ml sample is taken, and the remaining 190 ml is reinfused back.
5. The patient is ambulatory during the dwell time.
6. After 2 hours of dwell time, another sample of dialysis solution is taken and a blood sample is drawn.
7. After a 4 hour dwell time, the dialysis solution is drained out completely with the patient in a sitting position, the total volume is measured, and as sample is taken.
8. Concentration of creatinine and glucose are measured in the dialysis solution and blood samples. Glucose interferes with the Jaffe reagent for creatinine, thus creatinine values in the dialysis solution are overestimated. The correction factor in our laboratory is every mg/dl of glucose overestimates creatinine concentration by 0.0005 mg/dl. Creatinine values are corrected before any calculations are made.
9. Dialysate to plasma ratios (d/p) of creatinine at 2 and 4 hours and the ratios of dialysate glucose at 2 and 4 hours dwell time to dialysis solution glucose at 0 dwell time (d/d_0) are calculated.

2 PERITONEAL ACCESS

In the forties, Rosenak and Openheimer were the first to develop a specific peritoneal dialysis access. In the sixties, a rigid catheter made of polyvinyl chloride was introduced for acute peritoneal dialysis.

In 1964, Palmer and coworkers introduced the flexible silicone rubber peritoneal catheter which could be implanted and used repeatedly for lengthy periods of chronic peritoneal dialysis. Several modifications of the original Palmer catheter including the Tenckhoff catheter, are currently available for permanent implantation for chronic peritoneal dialysis (Figure 12).

Bedside access for acute peritoneal dialysis

The bedside insertion of a catheter becomes necessary when a patient with an acute renal failure is in an urgent need of dialysis. The bedside insertion technique is easy, and quickly accomplished.

A rigid catheter with multiple side holes is easily inserted at the bedside with the help of a sharp pointed stylet but needs frequent manipulation to maintain good function and, once inserted, can only be used safely for a maximum of 72 hours, beyond which the risk of peritonitis increases greatly.

Techniques of bedside catheter insertion and its associated complications are described in detail in the chapter dealing with acute renal failure.

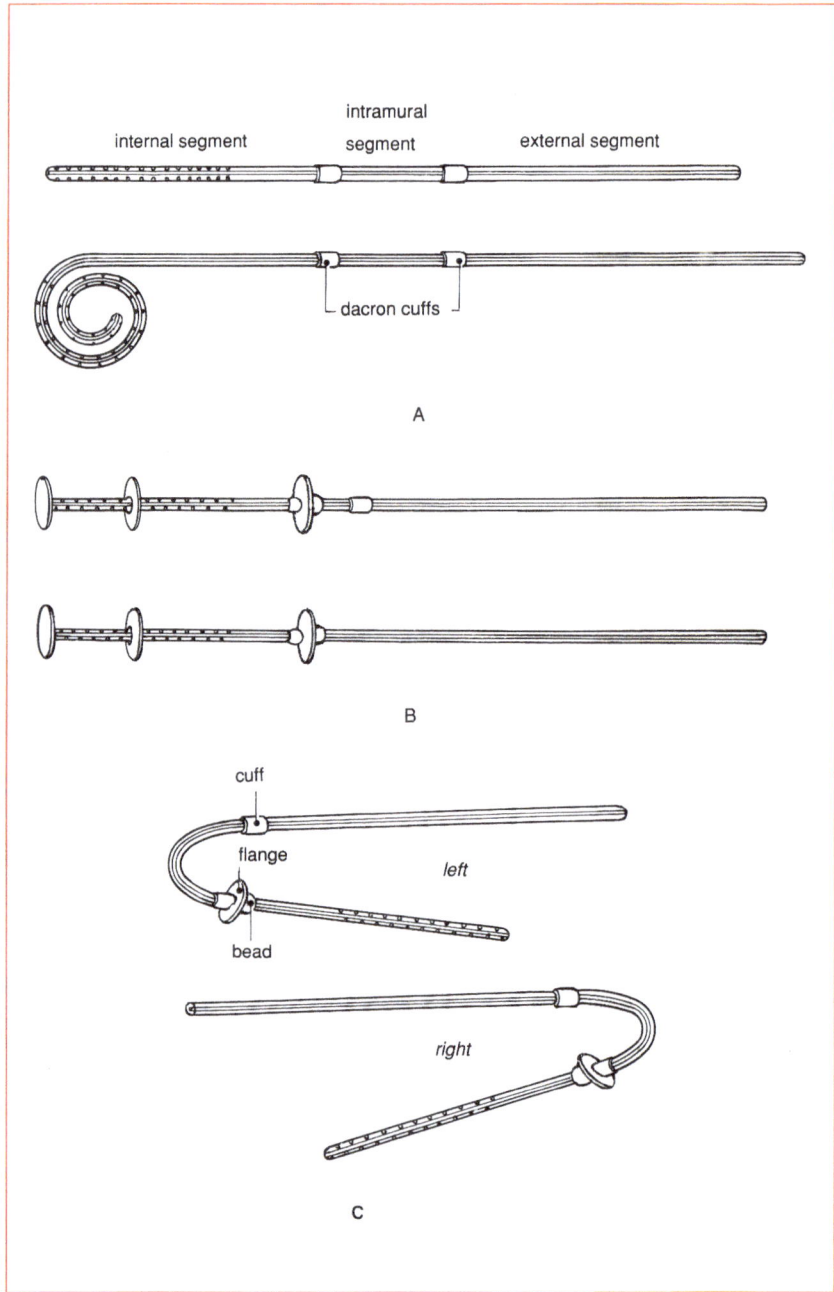

Figure 12: The Tenckhoff, Toronto Western Hospital (TWH), and Swan Neck Missouri catheters.

Long-term peritoneal access

The most widely used catheter for long-term use in patients on chronic peritoneal dialysis is the Tenckhoff catheter. This catheter, along with all its modified versions, is made of silicone rubber and has one or two cuffs made of Dacron velour (Figure 12). Silastic catheters are soft, flexible, atraumatic to the tissues, and biocompatible. The Dacron velour cuff permits profuse collagen tissue ingrowth between the fibers providing a strong bondage between it and the surrounding tissues. When implanted, the catheter is functionally recognized as having three segments: (a) an intraperitoneal segment with multiple side holes situated inside the peritoneal cavity for the inflow and outflow of the solution, (b) an intramural segment consisting of one or two cuffs, placed in the tunnel for catheter anchorage, to minimize dialysis solution leakage and to act as a barrier against the entry of bacteria into the peritoneum, and (c) an outer segment positioned outside the skin for easy connection for solution delivery. The differences between the Tenckhoff catheter and two of its most commonly

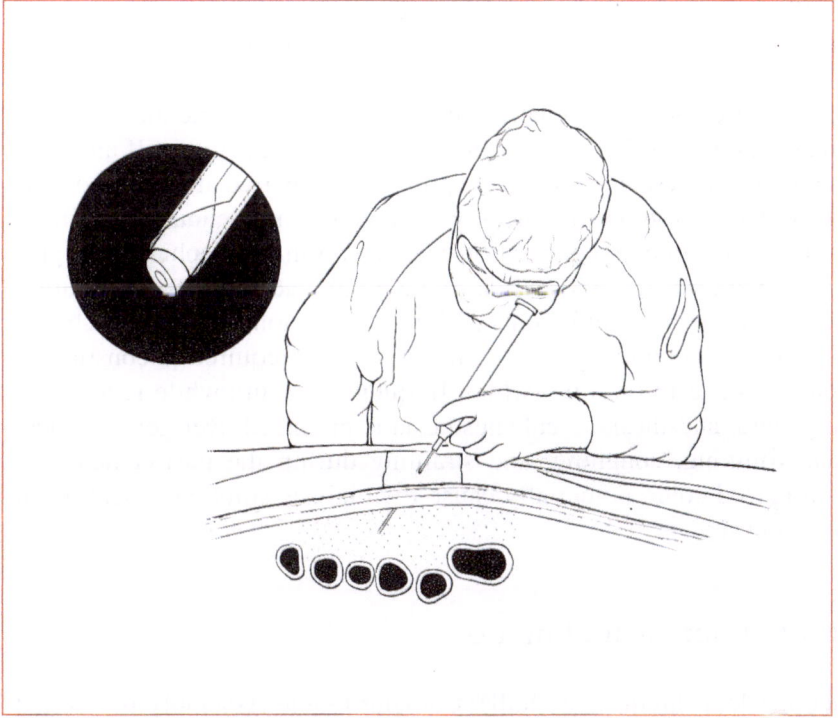

Figure 13: Peritoneal space is being viewed under direct vision through a Y-TEC® Scope. (Figure provided by and reproduced with permission of Medigroup, Inc., North Aurora, IL, USA.)

used modifications [Toronto Western (TWH) and Swan Neck Missouri (SNM) catheters] and the expected benefits of the modifications are given in Table 5.

Catheters for long-term use are implanted by an experienced surgeon in the operating room or nephrologist at the bedside.

The catheter insertion technique is variable from center to center and is greatly influenced by the local surgical practice. An experienced surgeon or a nephrologist with a special interest in peritoneal catheter implantation is a great asset to a peritoneal dialysis program.

The relative merits and shortcomings of some of the most commonly practiced techniques are summarized in Table 6.

Preinsertion patient preparation

The catheter insertion site and the desired location of the tunnel should be identified prior to implantation, taking into account the size and shape of the abdomen, the presence of previous surgical scars, belt line, and the patient's preference. Active peritonitis from previous acute dialysis must be treated and cured before implanting a permanent catheter. If an abdominal hernia is present, it should be preferably repaired at the time of catheter insertion. A gram of vancomycin is given intravenously within 24 hours to surgery or a first generation cephalosporin (i.e. cephalothin 1 gm) one or two hours prior to surgery is given prophylactically as a precaution against peri-operative infections. Prior to operation, the patient should empty the bladder and tap-water enemas may be required in constipated patients. To avert vomiting, which frequently occurs while recovering from general anesthesia, local anesthesia is preferred over general anesthesia. Vomiting, coughing, and straining during the post-catheter insertion period could potentially cause the dialysis solution to leak from the incision site.

Peritoneoscopic technique

Under sterile techniques, a Quill® Catheter Guide Assembly is inserted into the peritoneal cavity. After the intraperitoneal position of the assem-

® Medigroup, Inc., North Aurora, Illinois, USA.

TABLE 5. The differences between the Tenckhoff and the modified catheters [Toronto Western (TWH), and Swan neck (SNM)] and the expected benefits of the modifying features

	Tenckhoff	TWH	SNM	Expected benefits
Intraperitoneal segment	A segment with side holes.	A segment with side holes and two flat discs located at the terminal portion.	A segment with side holes.	The two flat discs of the TWH catheter helps to retain the inner segment in the pelvis.
Intramural segment	Straight 1 cm long outer and inner cuffs.	Straight 1 cm long outer and inner cuffs 1 cm diameter Dacron disc at the base of the inner cuff, placed perpendicular to the long axis of the catheter and a silicone bead with a groove between it and the disc.	N bend, 1 cm long outer and inner cuffs same as TWH except the disc is at a slanted angle.	The N bend of SNM helps (1) to retain the inner segment in the pelvis by providing a favorable tunnel direction like Tenckhoff and TWH catheters and (2) helps minimize exit-site infection through gravity drainage of debris from the sinus tract due to a caudally directed exit site. The Dacron disc and the silastic bubble in the TWH and SNM catheters allow the surgeon to position the catheter at the right place and, on healing, provides a firm bondage between the disc and the tissues to minimize dialysis solution leak. The slanted angle of SNM promotes the pelvic location of the inner segment.
External segment	similar in all three catheters.			

bly is confirmed through a Y-TEC® peritoneoscope (Figure 13), microfilter sterilized room air is insufflated into the peritoneal cavity. The cannula, with the surrounding Quill® catheter is dilated with a 7 French vascular dilator. Now the Tenckhoff catheter, stiffened with a flexible obturator, is inserted into the abdomen to the dilated Quill® catheter guide until the cuff is firmly seated amongst the abdominal musculature

TABLE 6. The merits and the shortcomings of different catheter insertion techniques

Bedside insertion techniques (Trocar and guidewire methods)

Merits:
1. Quick and convenient
2. Small incision
3. Immediate use possible with low risk of dialysis solution leakage
4. Due to the small incision low risk of late hernia
5. Low cost of the procedure

Shortcomings:
1. Blind procedure, and higher risk of early solution leakage
2. High risk of viscus perforation or tissue laceration
3. Inadequate hemostasis results in minor hemorrhages
4. Higher incidence of malfunction (poor flow)
5. Precise location of the inner segment may be difficult
6. Only Tenckhoff catheter insertion readily accomplished

Peritoneoscopic insertion

Merits:
1. Quick and convenient
2. Small incision; low risk of late hernias
3. Immediate use possible
4. Adequate hemostasis, low risk of bleeding
5. Lower risk of tissue injury
6. Precise positioning of the inner segment possible
7. Low cost, if done at the bedside

Shortcomings:
1. Expertise in using peritoneoscopy necessary
2. Only Tenckhoff catheter insertion possible

Surgical insertion technique

Merits:
1. Good hemostasis and low risk of bleeding
2. Tissue injury or viscus perforation is completely eliminated
3. Precise positioning of the inner segment is possible
4. All types of catheters can be inserted
5. Low risk of late dialysis solution leak with lateral/paramedian insertion

Shortcomings:
1. Larger incision may predispose to late hernias
2. Time taken for insertion is too long and in emergency situations could be a handicap
3. High cost of surgical procedure
4. Immediate use not recommended due to risk of dialysis solution leak through a larger
    incision

(Figures 33 A-C). The plastic Quill® catheter is carefully removed leaving the catheter and obturator in place. Now the obturator is removed. The external portion of the catheter is brought out through a subcutaneous tunnel. The steps of creating a subcutaneous tunnel are decribed on page 27.

Surgical technique

After surgical preparation of the abdomen, the skin over the incision and tunnel is anesthetized with 1% xylocaine. A 3–4 cm lateral paramedian transverse incision is made through the skin and through subcutaneous tissue (Figure 14A). Then, an incision is made in the anterior rectus sheath (Figure 14B) and the rectus muscle fibers are dissected bluntly down to the posterior rectus sheath. A purse-string suture is placed through the posterior rectus sheath, transversalis fascia, and through the peritoneum (Figure 14C). A 5 mm incision reaching the peritoneal cavity is made with a scalpel (Figure 14D). Care is used to protect the viscera from injury during this maneuver. The catheter is threaded on a wetted straight stiffening stylet and introduced deep into the true pelvis (Figure 14E). At this time, the patient may feel some pressure on the bladder or rectum. The radio-opaque stripe on the catheter is kept facing anteriorly. The stylet is removed, and then the patency of the catheter is tested by running in and immediately draining out a small volume of dialysis solution. A satisfactorily functioning catheter drains, on an average, at least 200 ml of solution in a minute. Slow drainage usually indicates an unsuitable location of the intraperitoneal segment or a faulty insertion technique, i.e. kinking, etc., in which case repositioning of the internal segment is necessary. If the solution flows freely, the internal cuff (in the case of Tenckhoff catheters) is brought into the field and the peritoneum is closed tightly with an absorbable suture under direct vision (Figure 14F). At this point, the cuff is laid longitudinally, parallel to the rectus muscle, and a stab wound is made in the anterior rectus fascia 3 cm cephalad to the transverse skin incision (Figure 14G). The external and intramural segments of the catheter is pulled through the fascia (Figure 14H). The transverse incision in the anterior rectus sheath is sutured (Figure 14I).

The catheter insertion through a paramedian incision via the rectus muscle is the currently preferred practice, although midline insertion is still preferred by some.

In the case of the Toronto Western Hospital and the Swan Neck Missouri catheters, the bead is placed in the peritoneal cavity, the flange on the posterior rectus sheath (Figure 15A) and the purse string suture is tightened

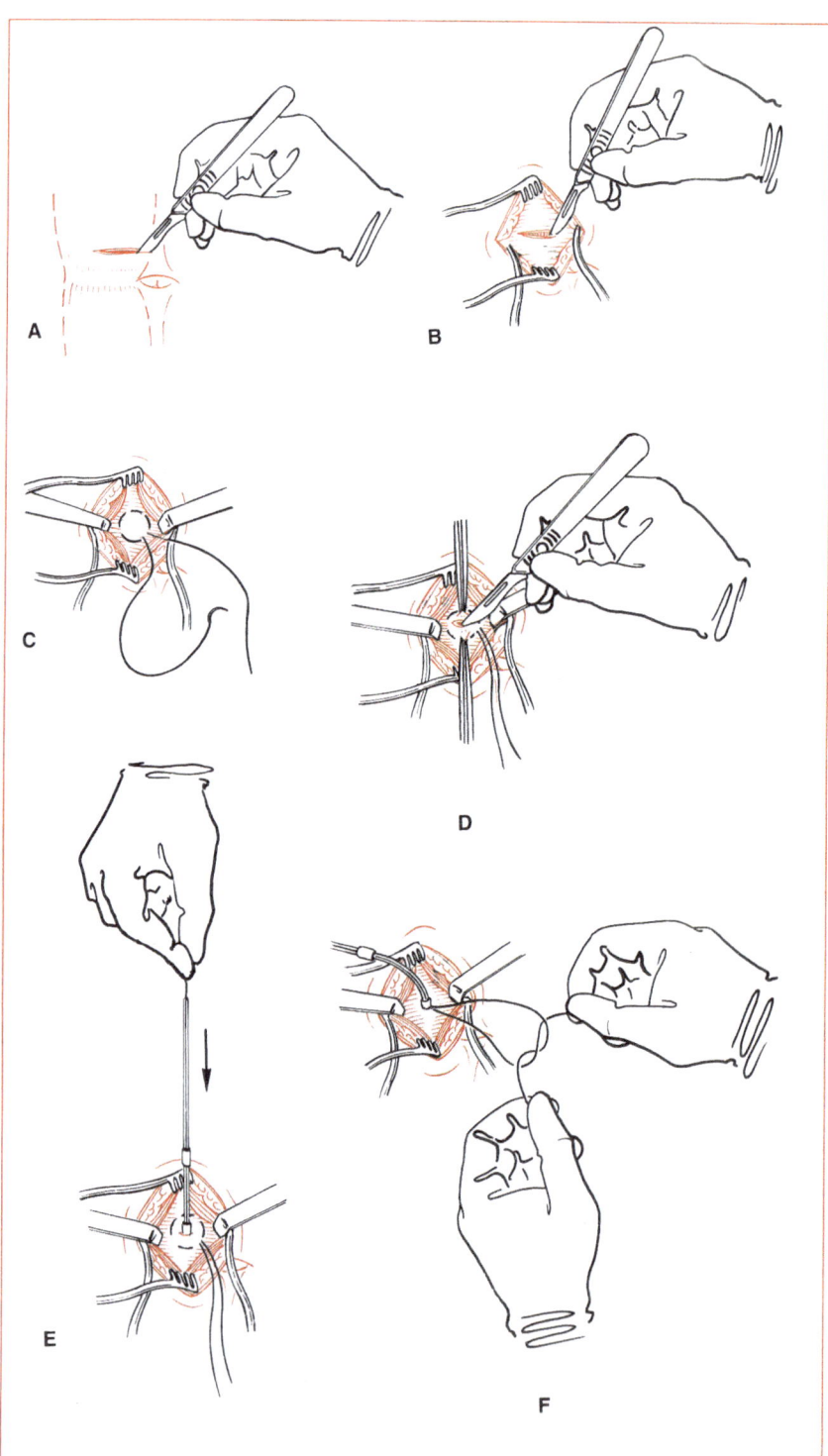

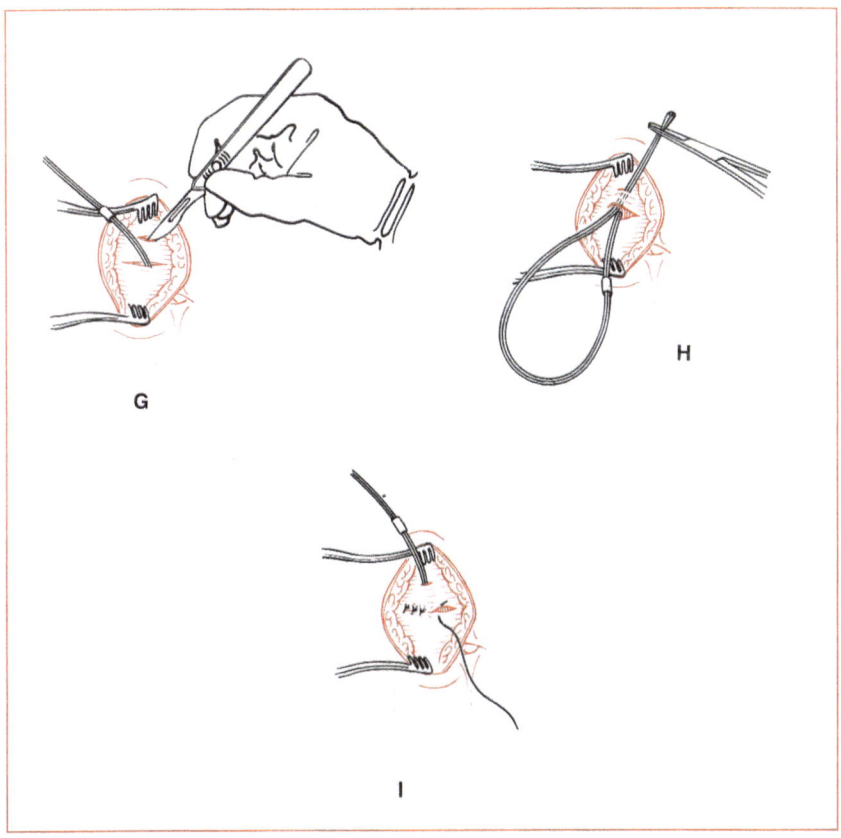

Figure 14: The steps of surgical insertion of the Tenckhoff catheter.

between them (Figure 15B). The flange is sewn to the posterior rectus with four sutures at twelve, nine, six, and three o'clock positions (Figure 15C).

Creation of a subcutaneous tunnel

The catheter tunnel extending from the cuff to the skin exit should have a diameter close to that of the catheter tubing. If the tunnel is too tight, it will not allow free drainage of necrotic tissue and may cause pressure necrosis with skin sloughing. On the other hand, a large tunnel prolongs healing relative to the volume of tissue required and allows movement of the catheter within the tunnel. This mechanical stress further delays the

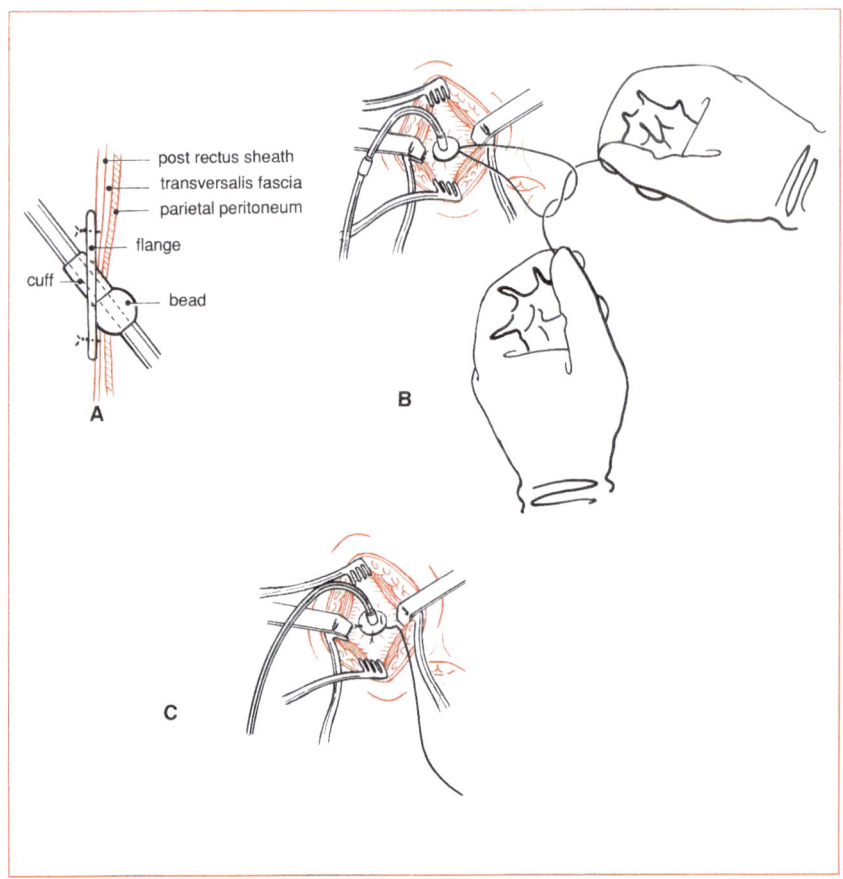

Figure 15A–C: The insertion technique of flange and bead in the Toronto Western Hospital and Swan Neck Missouri catheters.

healing process. Therefore, the sinus track should be made with a tunneler of an external diameter similar to that of the catheter tubing.

For Tenckhoff and TWH catheters, using a hemostat, a subcutaneous tunnel is made superior to the site suture on the rectus fascia (Figure 16A). The tunnel should be next to the abdominal wall musculature, deep to the subcutaneous tissue. A metal trocar is attached to the end of the catheter and the sharp end of the trocar is passed through the subcutaneous pocket and is brought out externally through a hole in the skin (Figure 16B). The external cuff is positioned at least 1 or 2 cm from the skin exit site (Figure 16C).

For the SNM catheter, a superior subcutaneous pocket is made to the level of skin markings to accommodate the bent portion of the catheter. The

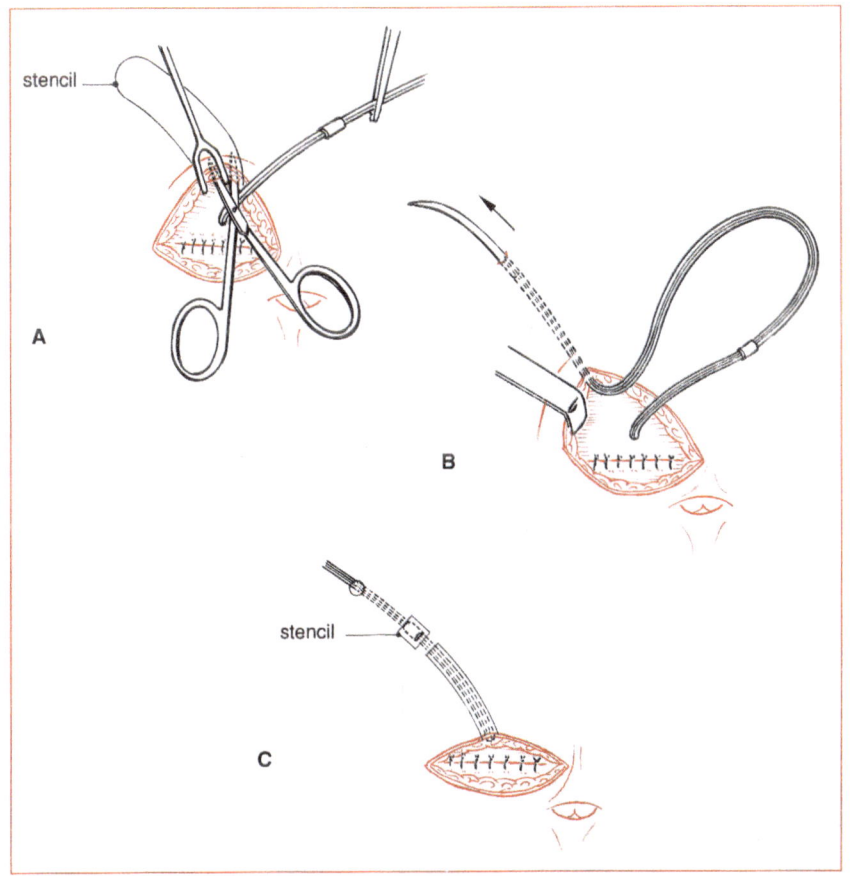

Figure 16A–C: Creation of a straight subcutaneous tunnel for the Tenckhoff and TWH catheters.

area between the subcutaneous pocket and the skin exit is anesthetized and the pocket is extended by blunt probing with the hemostat up to the point where the external cuff will lodge (Figure 17A). The bent portion of the catheter is carefully positioned in the subcutaneous pocket. A trocar is attached to the catheter and directed through the exit site (Figure 17B). The external cuff is positioned about 1 cm from the skin surface (Figure 17C). Care is taken to keep the radio-opaque stripe facing forwards.

The skin incision is closed with absorbable subcuticular sutures. The catheter is immobilized and the insertion site is covered with several layers of gauze dressing and secured with microfoam surgical tape. Care is taken to keep the radio-opaque stripe facing front. The dressing is left in place for a week unless a complication supervenes.

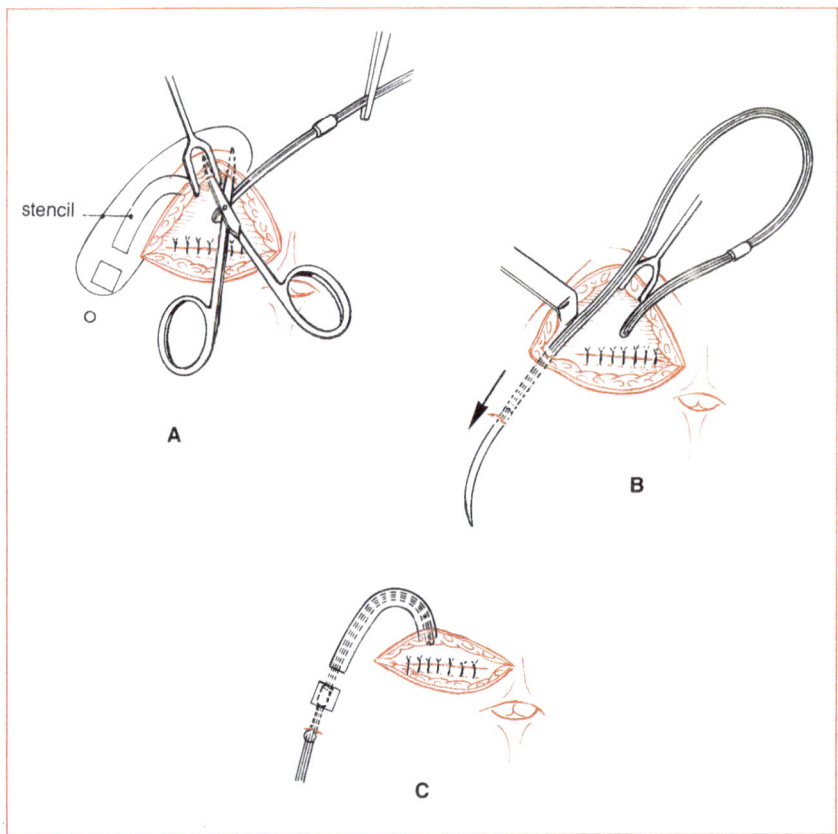

Figure 17A–C: Creation of a subcutaneous tunnel for the Swan Neck Missouri catheter.

Post-operative care

The external end of the catheter is connected to a transfer set through a titanium adapter. Additional in-and-out exchanges are performed with 1 liter of dialysis solution to remove residual blood from the peritoneal cavity, if present. The position of the catheter segment in the peritoneal cavity is documented by a plain X-ray of the abdomen. This information could be useful should a flow problem occur in the future.

Frequently, a catheter may function poorly due to constipation. Analgesics (opiates) causing constipation should be avoided in the post-operative period. Drainage is usually slow (<150 ml/min) if the catheter tip is not in the true pelvis. A migrated internal segment does not always result in functional inadequacy. If the position of the internal catheter segment is not in the true pelvis, no immediate surgical correction is attempted, even if the catheter function is inadequate. Spontaneous relocation to the pelvic cavity with a return of adequate function may occur within a few days. In the interim, empirically, the patient may be given a laxative in an attempt to force the relocation. Failure to relocate after a reasonable observation period may compel a surgical repositioning. A persistently nonfunctioning catheter with the internal segment in the true pelvis is an indication of the omental capture of the catheter. For correction, surgical repositioning with or without omentectomy may be necessary.

Certain conditions such as diabetes, obesity, debilitating chronic illness, and steroid treatment in the period immediately prior to catheter insertion, are usually associated with poor wound healing and may predispose to a dialysis solution leakage if they are started on standard volume peritoneal dialysis. In such patients, the initial exchange volume should be as low as possible, i.e., 500–1000 ml per exchange. Initiation of CAPD with the standard volume of dialysis solution should be delayed until wound healing has taken place. Peritoneal dialysis in the supine position may be given if necessary. Alternatively, such patients may be given hemodialysis through a subclavian catheter until the patient is ready to resume CAPD.

Catheter break-in

The break-in period for a peritoneal catheter follows catheter insertion. During the healing period, undue stress exerted on the incision by the high intra-abdominal pressure with 2 liters of dialysis solution (especially in the upright position) may disrupt the healing process and cause dialysis solution leakage. Leakage not only delays ingrowth of fibrous tissue into the cuffs, but also provides a medium for bacterial growth, thus increasing the risk of peritonitis and exit-site infection. It is therefore desirable to delay initiation of standard CAPD for at least 10–15 days after catheter implantation.

> To minimize complications, strict adherence to the break-in procedure is essential. The steps suggested in the break-in procedure allow sufficient time for the incision to heal before standard CAPD is begun, at the same time taking care to maintain the catheter patency.

Catheters inserted at the bedside usually require no break-in period although some physicians use reduced volume (500 ml, then 1000 ml) for the initial four to eight exchanges before proceeding to the normal 2000 ml exchange volume (in patients with a small abdomen or with respiratory embarrassment, a reduced exchange volume may be required indefinitely).

In ESRD patients when a catheter is inserted for long-term use, the catheter may be used for initial acute dialysis in the supine position because the intra-abdominal pressure during filling in the supine position is limited and leakage is not usually a problem. A liter volume is used for the first session of supine peritoneal dialysis. If a cycler is used, the usual cycler settings are 5–6 min inflow, 10 min dwell, and 10 min outflow. Heparin (500–1000 units per liter of dialysis sulution) may be added to facilitate free flow. Several sessions of supine dialysis may be given until the incision is well healed and ready to commence standard CAPD.

When a catheter is replaced in a patient who is already on CAPD, provide peritoneal dialysis only in the supine position with a cycler until the incision is well healed. Alternatively, hemodialysis is provided using a subclavian or internal jugular vein catheter as an access until standard CAPD can be resumed.

At the time of catheter insertion, another abdominal surgery, such as hernia repair, cholecystectomy, etc., is performed, and no change in break-in procedure is recommended except that standard CAPD may be delayed for longer than 15 days depending on the surgeon's recommendation.

Subsequent catheter care

The surgical dressing placed at the time of insertion is removed after one week. Care is taken to avoid catheter pulling or twisting. The exit and skin surrounding the catheter are cleansed with hydrogen peroxide and liquid soap, rinsed with sterile water, patted dry with sterile gauze, covered with several layers of gauze dressings, and secured with microfoam surgical tape. Weekly dressing changes are continued until the healing process is completed, which may be up to 6 weeks. Patients may take sponge baths.

> Special precautions, such as routine cleaning and dressing, and avoidance of trauma, etc., of the exit site, after the healing process is completed, are essential to prevent infection.

The catheters should be anchored in such a way that the patient's movements are only minimally transmitted to the exit. The method of catheter immobilization is individualized, depending on exit location and shape of abdomen.

> Protection of the catheter from mechanical stress is extremely important, more so during the break-in period.

Exit-site care

Special care of the exit site after the healing process is completed is essential to prevent infection. Routine exit-site care after good healing includes (1) frequent examination (once or twice a week) by the patient of the exit-site and tunnel for signs of infection, (2) daily or alternate-day cleaning of the skin to remove dirt, and (3) immobilization of the catheter to avoid tension and trauma. Following satisfactory healing (6–8 weeks after implantation) besides showering, swimming pools (preferably after covering the exit site, catheter spike, and dialysate bag with a colostomy bag) may be permitted. Tub-bathing should be avoided.

The complications in the early period after surgical insertion are similar to those after acute catheter insertion except their occurrence rates are considerably lower.

> When catheters are implanted with strict adherence to steps of insertion, the incidence of early and late complications are very low. Over the long-term, exit-site infection is the major problem related to peritoneal access. The other late complications, namely, dialysis solution leak, poor in-and-out flow, and cuff extrusion occur very infrequently.

Dialysis-solution leakage may occur months or even years after catheter insertion. Most cases of late dialysis-solution leakage are refractory to conservative management, such as stopping peritoneal dialysis for a few weeks or switching to supine dialysis with lower volume exchanges, and require surgical repair. External cuff extrusion is a late complication usually due to the placement of (1) the superficial cuff at a distance of less than 1 cm from the skin exit site, and (2) the intramural catheter segment in a shape other than the natural shape. Late catheter malfunction (poor drainage, etc.) is extremely uncommon and when it occurs, is usually in association with severe peritonitis.

The problem of exit-site infection is discussed in detail in another chapter.

Indications for catheter removal

Catheters may have to be removed
   (1) if they function poorly, or
   (2) if their presence in the peritoneal cavity may promote peritonitis or delay the response to appropriate therapy, or
   (3) when they are no longer needed.

Poor functioning or nonfunctioning catheters may be removed under the following conditions:

(1) persistent intraluminal obstruction from any cause,
(2) internal segment migration out of the pelvis with persistent poor flow,
(3) a catheter kink along its course,
(4) a catheter with its intraperitoneal segment caught in adhesions following severe peritonitis.

A functioning catheter may have to be removed under the following conditions:

(1) recurrent peritonitis without an identifiable cause,
(2) peritonitis due to exit-site and/or tunnel infections,
(3) persistent exit-site and/or tunnel infection,
(4) late recurrent dialysis solution leak through the exit site or into the layers of the abdominal wall,
(5) unusual peritonitis, i.e. tuberculous, fungal, etc.,
(6) bowel perforation with fecal peritonitis,
(7) refractory peritonitis,
(8) persistent severe abdominal pain either due to the catheter impinging on internal organs or during solution inflow, and
(9) catheter cuff erosion with infection.

3 TECHNIQUES, PRESCRIPTIONS, AND INDICATIONS

Current techniques of peritoneal dialysis utilize infusion and, after a variable dwell period, drainage of the dialysis solution through the indwelling peritoneal catheter. Volume describes the amount of dialysis solution used per exchange and dose depicts the amount of solution used over a specified time period. The terms intermittent (periodic treatment interspersed between periods with no treatment) and continuous (treatment given 24 hours a day, 7 days a week with no interruptions) peritoneal dialysis describe regimens or plans of therapy over a period of time. A prescription includes the method of dialysis (manual or machine), regimen (intermittent or continuous), infusion volume, and dose of dialysis. Categorization of the peritoneal membrane based on the peritoneal equilibration test is helpful in predicting the appropriate dialysis regimen for a given patient (Figure 18).

Intermittent regimens

Intermittent regimens are especially suitable for patients who have significant residual renal function and/or high peritoneal transport rates (Figures 19).

Daytime Ambulatory Peritoneal Dialysis (DAPD): Treatment is given during the day for 12–16 hours, when the patient is ambulatory, and not during the night. The duration of each exchange is no more than three to four hours. The patient with a high peritoneal equilibration rate will generate sufficient net ultrafiltration to maintain a good fluid balance and the short exchange time will allow the capture of peak clearances of small solutes.

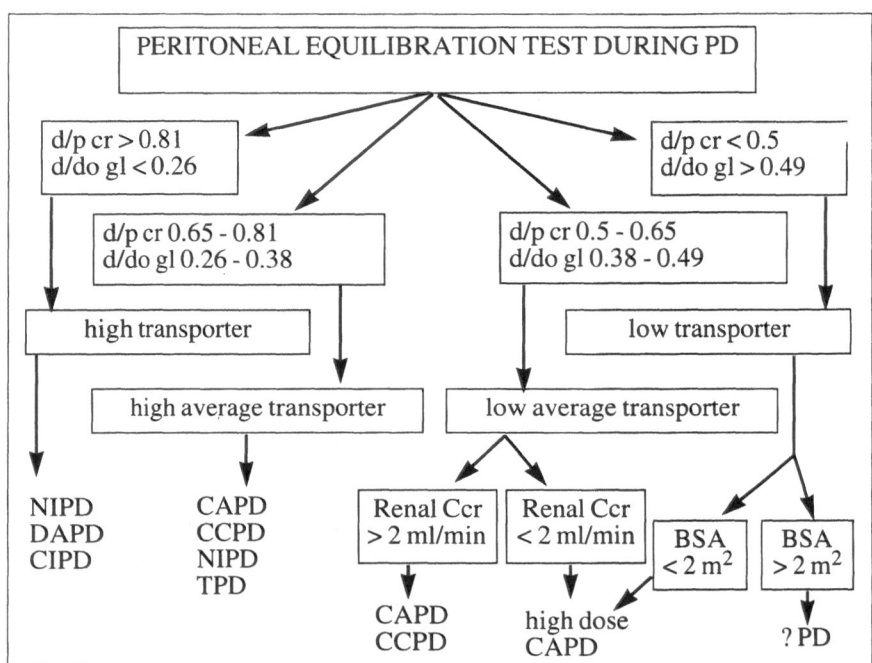

Figure 18: Choosing a PD regimen based on the peritoneal membrane equilibration rate. NIPD = Nightly intermittent PD,   CAPD = Continuous ambulation PD
DAPD = Daytime ambulatory PD, CCPD = Continuous cyclic PD
CIPD = Chronic intermittent PD,   TPD = Tidal PD
BSA = Body Surface Area,   Ccr = Creatinine Clearance

Intermittent peritoneal Dialysis (IPD): Treatment is given over a 20 hour period with the help of a cycler machine, twice a week. Between treatments, the peritoneal cavity is empty. A high or high average peritoneal equilibration rate patient is the most suitable for such a regimen. The dose per session is usually 40–60 liters. A patient with an average rate of small solute clearance can be adequately dialyzed with this regimen provided he or she has a significant residual renal function.

Nightly Intermittent Peritoneal Dialysis (NIPD): Treatment is given with the help of a cycler every night while the patient sleeps, lasting for 8–12 hours. The daytime is free of treatment. The dose is usually 15–20 liters. To provide adequate dialysis with a shorter (8–10 hours) treatment session, the patient may have to use one or two daytime exchanges. The volume of the daytime exchange may be tailored to the patient's condition, i.e. a patient with a hernia may tolerate no more than an 800–1000 ml volume.

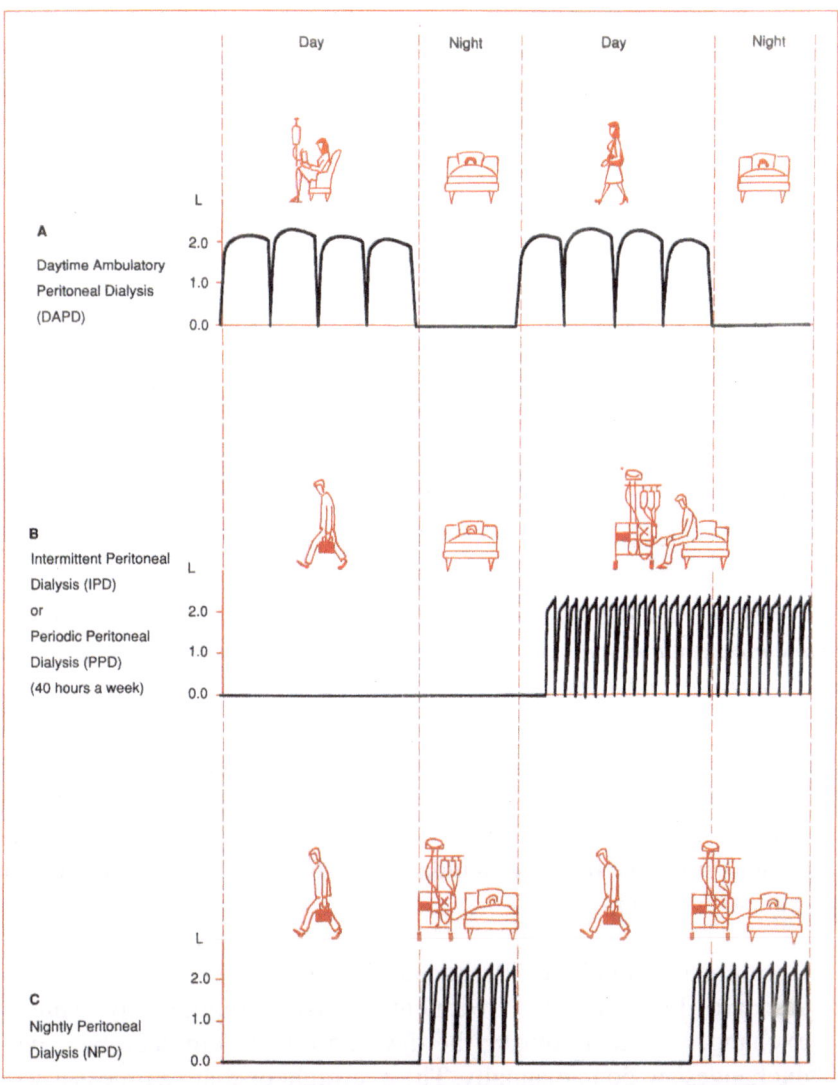

Figure 19: Intermittent regimens of peritoneal dialysis. These regimens allows the patient to be free of dialysis for a specified period in between the dialysis treatments. The exchanges are done manually as in DAPD or with the help of a cycler as in IPD or NPD. A: DAPD, B: IPD, C: NPD.

Continuous regimens

Continuous ambulatory peritoneal dialysis (CAPD) and continuous cyclic peritoneal dialysis (CCPD) are the two continuous regimens (Figure 20). In standard CAPD/CCPD, 2 liter volumes are used per exchange.

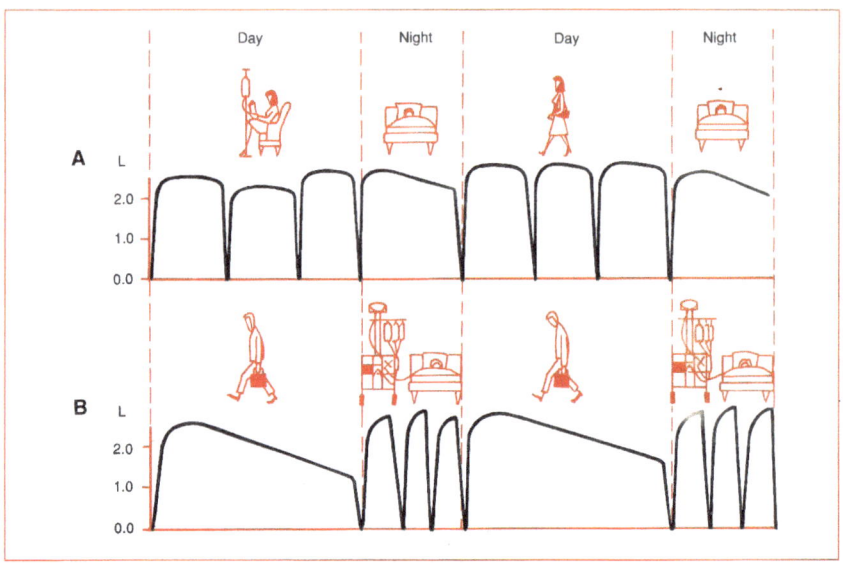

*Figure 20: Continuous regimens of dialysis. The dialysis exchanges are perform-
ed at convenient times, and the dialysis solution is in the peritoneal cavity all the
time to provide continuous dialysis. A = CAPD, B = CCPD.*

During CAPD, three manual exchanges are usually performed during the
day and one during the night. During CCPD, exchanges are performed
with the help of a cycler; three during the night and one long dwell
exchange during the day. The standard dose for CAPD/CCPD for an adult
patient is 7.5–9 liters per day.

Continuous Ambulatory Peritoneal Dialysis (standard volume and
standard dose CAPD): Treatment is given continuously. Three
exchanges are done during the day and one before bedtime. The
exchanges are done manually. The overnight exchange time is usually 8–10 hours. The glucose concentration of the overnight
exchange is chosen according to the patient's ultrafiltration need
and peritoneal membrane equilibration rate. The amount of fluid
absorbed during a long overnight exchange can be significant,
especially in a patient with a high solute equilibration rate, in which
case a higher glucose concentration solution should be selected. A
patient with an average or a high peritoneal equilibration rate is the
ideal candidate for this treatment.

Continuous Cyclic Peritoneal Dialysis (standard volume, standard
dose CCPD): Treatment is given continuously. The three nightly

exchanges are done with the help of a cycler. The duration of the one long daytime exchange is 14–16 hours. The patient best suited for CAPD can also do CCPD but the need of a partner to help with the treatment requires him or her to choose CCPD. Infants, school children, and elderly debilitated patients requiring support are those who choose CCPD over CAPD.

Alternate PD regimens

For adequate dialysis, a patient with a low average or low solute equilibration rate requires more dialysis. Since CAPD and CCPD are continuous treatments, prescriptions can only be modified by changing the volume per exchange and/or dose per day. Such modifications, although they provide adequate dialysis, are not practical because of the significant time required to perform manual dialysis. IPD and NIPD prescriptions are modified not only by increasing the dose of the treatment and/or the volume of an exchange, but also by increasing the time of the treatment. Patients accept and adapt to a treatment time of 10–12 hours per day because such treatment is carried out during sleeping time. However, increasing the treatment time beyond 10–12 hours a day may not be a practical solution. Some alternate PD regimens are described in Figure 21.

Standard dose, high volume CAPD: The dose of dialysis per day is maintained at 7.5–9 liters but the volume of exchange is increased to over 2 liters. This option may be attractive to some patients who work during the day.

High dose, standard volume CAPD: The dose of dialysis per day exceeds 9 liters while maintaining the 2-liter volume per exchange. This will require the patient to perform more than 4 exchanges per day. Suitable for patients who are unable to tolerate higher volumes per exchange due to predisposition, to hernia, or to cardiorespiratory difficulties.

High dose, high volume CAPD: Volume per exchange is more than 2 liters and the dose per day is more than 9 liters. Suitable for anuric patients with a high body surface area and low solute equilibration rates.

High dose CCPD I: Total dose of dialysis exceeds 9 liters per day mainly by increasing the duration of the nightly phase (>8 hours) of

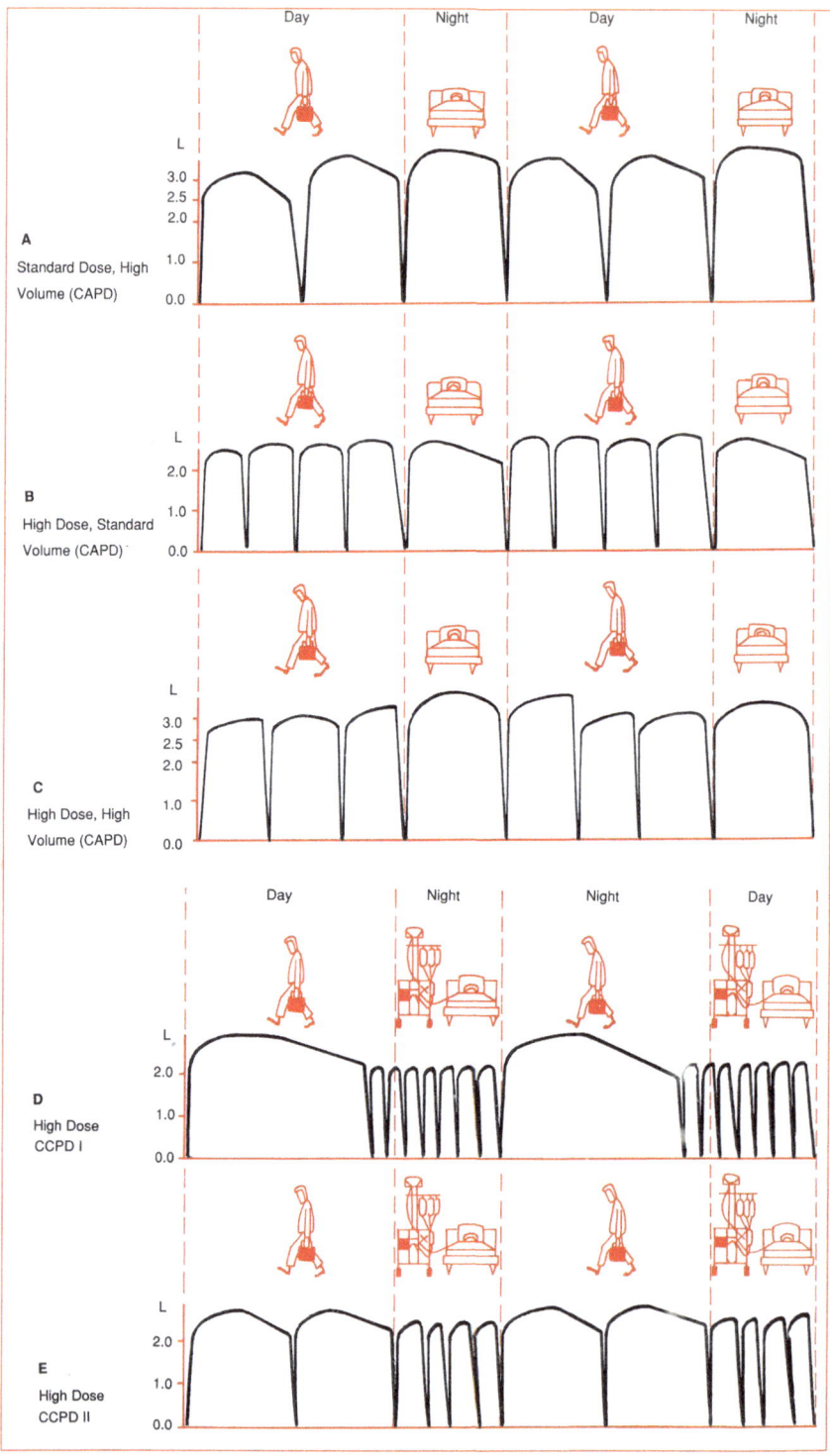

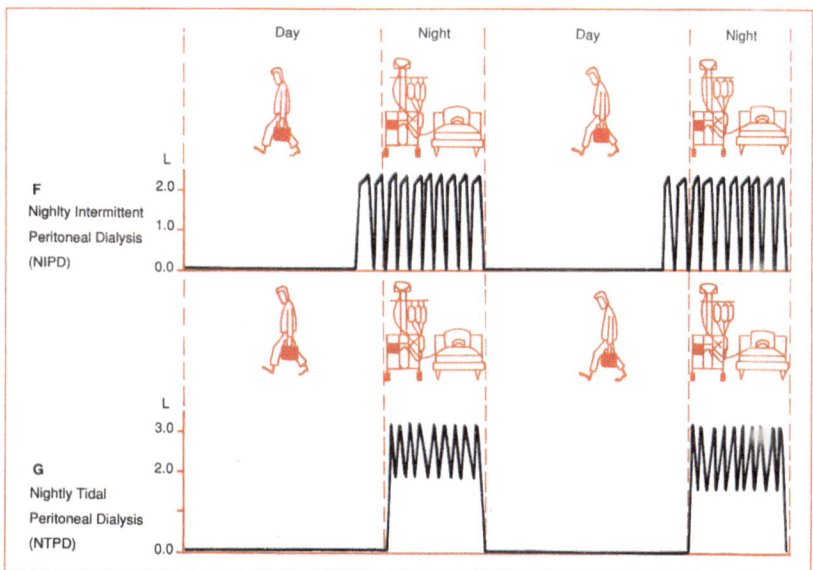

Figure 21: Alternate PD regimens. The dose per session or day, volume per exchange, and timings of the treatment are adjusted to the patient's convenience. A: standard dose, high volume CAPD; B: high dose, standard volume CAPD; C: high dose, high volume CAPD; D: high dose CCPD I; E: high dose CCPD II; F: high dose NIPD; G: nightly TPD.

dialysis and dose over 8 liters but continue to perform one single daytime exchange with a 2-liter volume.

High dose CCPD II: The dialysis dose is increased by performing more than one exchange during the daytime. Nightly cycler-based exchanges remain similar to the standard prescription or may be increased.

High dose nightly intermittent peritoneal dialysis (NIPD): In an anuric patient, a typical dialysis session lasts for 10–12 hours. A typical dose of dialysis solution per session is about 20–24 liters.

Nightly tidal peritoneal dialysis (NTPD): In the tidal flow technique, a constant volume (1200–1500 ml) of dialysis solution (reserve volume) is maintained in the peritoneal cavity throughout the treatment session. Over and above this reserve volume, rapid exchanges are carried out with the help of a cycler infusing a fixed tidal volume (1000–1500 ml) of dialysis solution. For adequate dialysis in an anuric patient, typically a session of dialysis lasts about 8–10 hours. A typical dose is about 30–36 liters per session.

The CAPD and home cycler therapies have their unique medical and psychosocial advantages and disadvantages which are listed in Table 7.

The indications for CAPD/CCPD treatment are listed in Table 8A.The indications for CCPD over CAPD are given in Table 8B. Since treatment has both a medical and psychosocial impact on a patient's medical condition and life style, these factors should be taken into consideration when individualizing a dialysis prescription.

TABLE 7. CAPD compared to home cycler peritoneal dialysis

	Standard CAPD 40-50 liter/weekof C_{Cr}	Home cycler PD 40-50 liter/weekof C_{Cr}
Medical:		
Weekly clearances	Adequate	Adequate
Sodium removal	Usually sufficient	May be insufficient
Thirst mechanism	Normal	Stimulated
Blood pressure	Easily normalized	May be high
Blood chemistries	Steady	Fluctuating
Peritonitis rate	Higher	Low
Metabolic problems	Obesity, hyperlipidemia	Hyperlipidemia
High IP pressure	Hernias, hemorrhoids dialysis solution leak, low back pain	Less frequent
Psychosocial:		
Equipments	Simple	Complex machines
Travel	Easy	Difficult
Bed confined	No	Prolonged
Body image	Distorted	Normal
Day activities	Interrupted	Uninterrupted
Compliance	Frequent noncompliance	Good

TABLE 8A. Indications for CCPD and CAPD
(Modified from Hamburger et al., Dialysis and Transplantation 1990; 19:66)

Medical	Demographic	Psychosocial
PREFERRED (strongly indicated) for CAPD:		
- Vascular access difficult to (establish) - Transfusion problem (X-match or Jehovah's Witness) - Preservation of residual renal function - Refractory heart failure	- Age 0–5 years	- Long way from center - Strong patient preference - Strong need for autonomy independence or control
INDICATED for CAPD:		

- Diabetes mellitus
- Cardiovascular disease
  - Angina
  - Prosthetic valvular disease
  - Arrhythmias
  - Valvular heart disease
- Chronic disease
  - Anemia (symptomatic or transfusion dependent)
  - HIV positive
  - Known bleeding disorder
  - Hepatitis
  - Peripheral vascular disease
  - Hemosiderosis
- Transplant candidates
	- All ages
	- Both sexes
	- All races
		- Active life styles
		- Variable schedule
		- Travel
		- Needle anxiety
		- Demand for flexible die

VARIABLY INDICATED for CAPD:		
- Obesity/large size - COPD - Polycystic kidney disease - History of diverticulitis - Low back pain - Recurrent hernias - Multiple abdominal surgery - Blindness - Impaired manual dexterity - Scleroderma - Steroid therapy - Chronic recurrent pancreatitis - Lupus	- Nursing home	- Severe depression - Drug abuse - Social support needed
QUESTIONABLY INDICATED for CAPD:		
- Malnutrition - Multiple abdominal adhesions - Ostomies - Hiatal hernia with reflux esophagitis - Severe diabetic gasproparesis - Severe hypertriglyceridemia	- Homeless - Transplant within one month	- Chronic poor - Poor compliance - Dementia
CONTRAINDICATED for CAPD:		

- Severe inflammatory bowel disease
  - Acute active diverticulitis
  - Active ischemic bowel disease
  - Abdominal abscess
- Low peritoneal membrane transport
		- Severe active psychotic or depressive disorder
		- Marked intellectual disability with no helper

TABLE 8B. Indications for CCPD over CAPD

Medical:
1. Patients with complications related to raised IP pressure i.e. hernias, fluid leaks, hemorrhoids, back pain, etc.
2. Inadequate small solute clearances
3. Inadequate ultrafiltration
4. Frequent peritonitis episodes during CAPD

Psychosocial:
1. School children
2. Employed active patients
3. Helper convenience
4. Poor body image
5. Poor compliance

(Illustrations and glossaries used in this chapter are adapted from Twardowski, Zbylut J. Peritoneal dialysis glossary III. In: Peritoneal Dialysis International 1990; 6:47–9.)

4 DIALYSIS SOLUTIONS AND EQUIPMENT

Dialysis solution

Dialysis solutions for CAPD are available in different glucose concentrations (0.5, 1.5, 2.5, and 4.25 g% of monohydrate glucose) and volumes (0.25, 0.5, 0.75, 1.0, 2.0, 2.5, and 3 liters) packaged in clear under-filled plastic bags of potential volume almost 50% more than the solution volume. The electrolyte concentrations of the solutions simulate normal serum values (Table 9). Because of the technical difficulties in the preparation and storage of a bicarbonate-containing solution, peritoneal dialysis solutions contain lactate as a bicarbonate generating agent.

TABLE 9. Composition of peritoneal dialysis solutions

	Solution 1	Solution 2	Solution 3
Sodium (mEq/l)	132	132	132
Magnesium (mEq/l)	1.5	0.5	0.5
Chloride	102	96	95
Calcium	3.5	3.5	2.5
Lactate	35	40	40
Dextrose		(1.5, 2.5, or 4.25 gm/dl)[a]	
pH	5.5	5.5	5.5

[a] Molecular weight of monohydrate d-glucose is about 10% greater than that of anhydrous glucose. Therefore, the true concentrations of glucose in solutions are 1.36, 2.27, or 3.86 gm/dl.

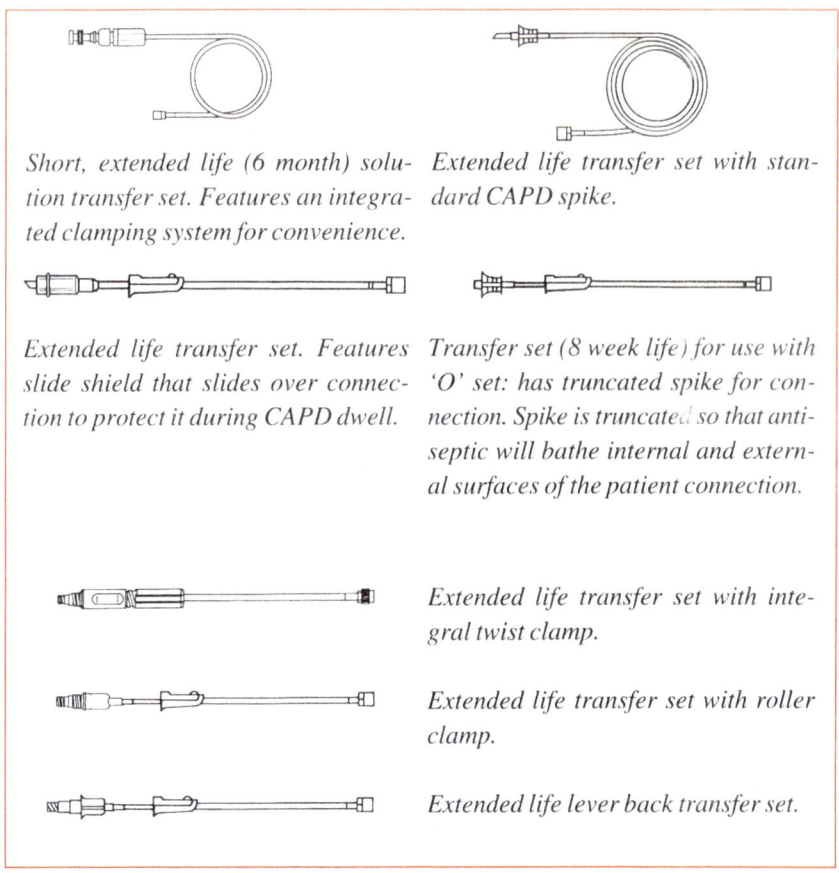

Short, extended life (6 month) solu-   *Extended life transfer set with stan-*
tion transfer set. Features an integra-   *dard CAPD spike.*
ted clamping system for convenience.

Extended life transfer set. Features   *Transfer set (8 week life) for use with*
slide shield that slides over connec-   *'O' set: has truncated spike for con-*
tion to protect it during CAPD dwell.   *nection. Spike is truncated so that anti-*
  septic will bathe internal and extern-
  al surfaces of the patient connection.

Extended life transfer set with inte-
gral twist clamp.

Extended life transfer set with roller
clamp.

Extended life lever back transfer set.

Figure 22: Straight transfer sets.

Transfer sets

The dialysis solution is infused from the plastic bags into the peritoneum through an indwelling catheter. The transfer set connects the solution bag with the catheter. It may be straight (Figure 22) or Y shaped (Figure 23). At one end of the straight transfer set is a spike for connection to the bag outlet port and at the other end is a Luer-lock connector for connection with the catheter. Added antiseptic protection may be obtained at the spike-outlet port connection site by using a connection shield containing a sponge soaked with povidone-iodine (Figure 24). It also locks the connection spike into the bag outlet port.

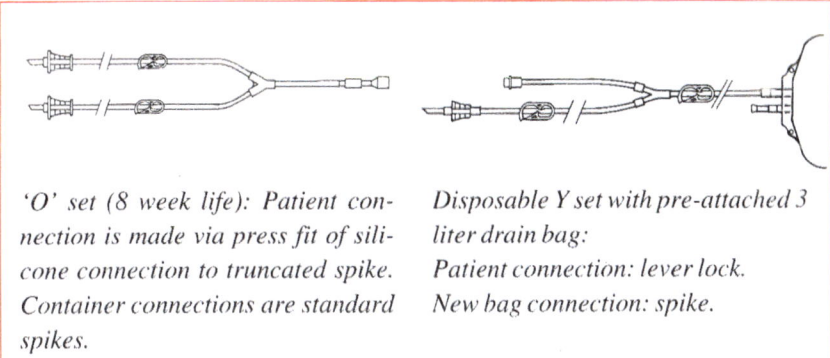

'O' set (8 week life): Patient connection is made via press fit of silicone connection to truncated spike. Container connections are standard spikes.

Disposable Y set with pre-attached 3 liter drain bag:
Patient connection: lever lock.
New bag connection: spike.

Figure 23: Y shaped transfer sets.

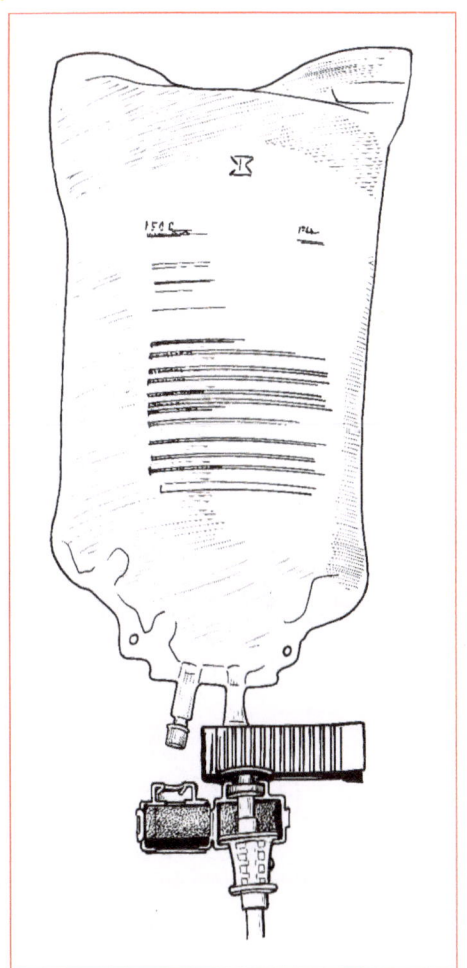

Figure 24: Connection site (spike-bag outlet port) is protected by a connection shield with a sponge soaked in povidone-iodine.

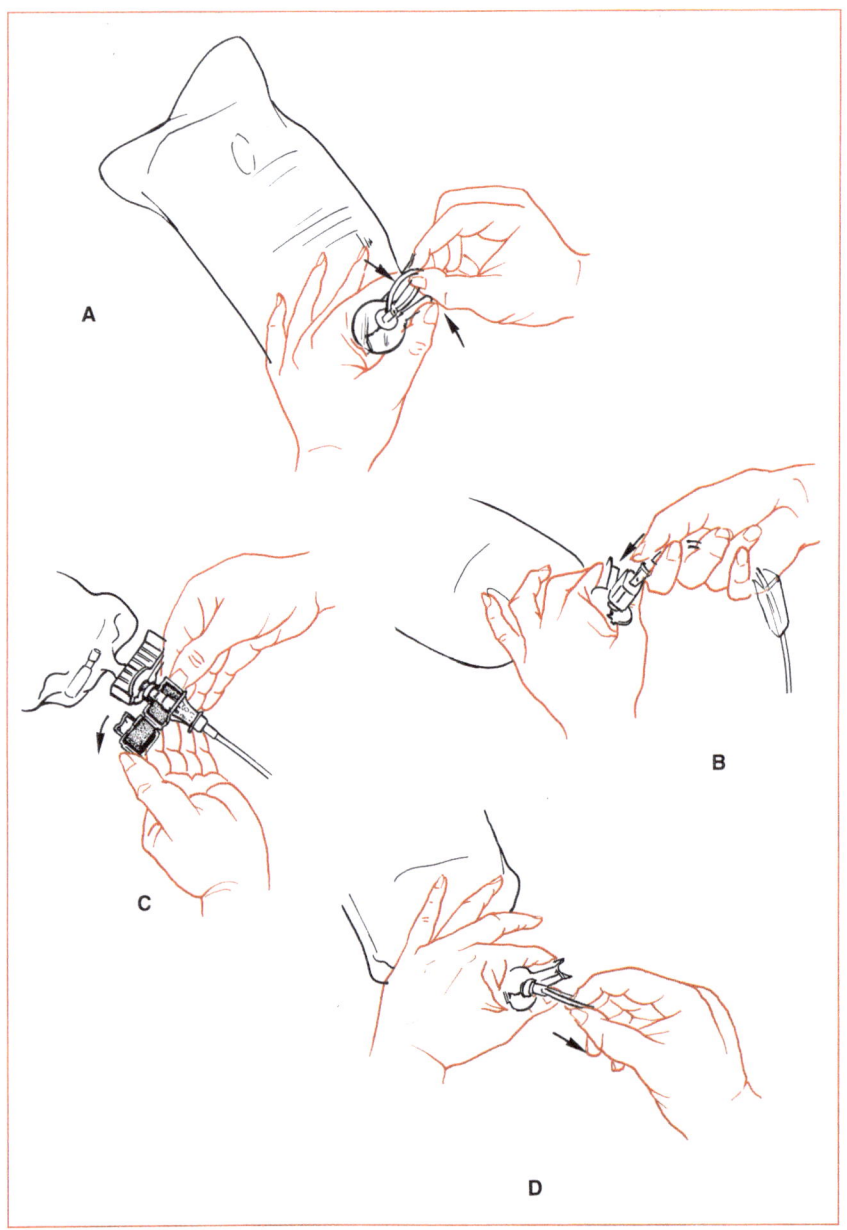

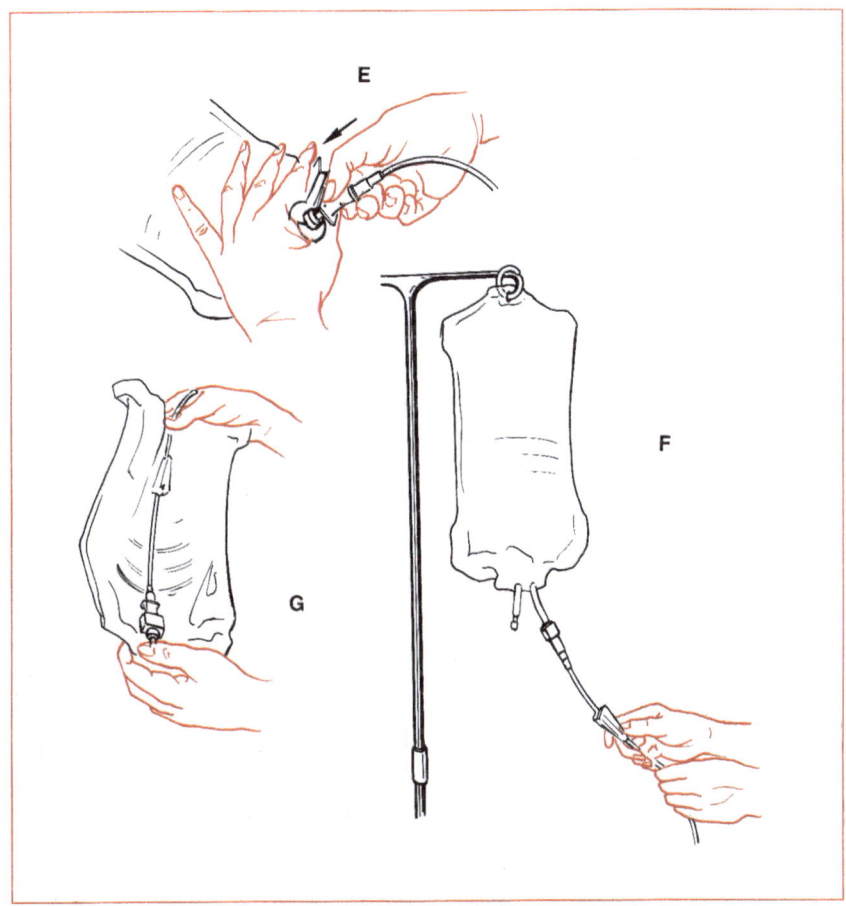

Figure 25: Steps of a solution exchange with a straight transfer set.

(A) Tape the injection port to the bag. Put an outlet port clamp on the port of the new bag close to the flange, leaving a small space.

(B) Put an outlet port clamp on the used bag directly behind the green connection shield. Be sure both bag ports hang over the edge of your work surface.

(C) Remove the connection shield from the used bag and discard it.

(D) Remove the pull ring from the outlet port of the new bag. Do not touch the port.

(E) Immediately spike the new bag. Do this step carefully. The shoulder of the spike should be even with the end of the port.

(F) Hang the new bag. Open the roller clamp and begin filling.

(G) When filling is over, close the roller clamp. Remove the bag from the fill position and fold it so that it can be worn comfortably. Throw away used supplies.

Steps of a solution exchange with a straight transfer set

During the manual solution exchange procedure, the dialysis solution is drained from the peritoneal cavity and discarded, and a new bag of peritoneal solution is infused by gravity into the peritoneal cavity. The entire procedure is carried out under an aseptic condition in a clean environment as follows: After masking, hands are washed. The empty bag from under the patient's clothes is placed in the drain position. After inspecting the new bag of solution for clarity and leaks, the injection port of the bag is taped and an outlet port clamp is put on the port of the new bag close to the flange, leaving a small opening (Figure 25A). When drainage is over, the roller clamp on the transfer set is closed. An outlet port clamp is put on the used bag directly behind the connection shield (Figure 25B). The connection shield is removed from the used bag and discarded Figure 25C). Without touching the port, the ring from the outlet port of the new bag is removed (Figure 25D). The spike from the used bag is removed without contaminating it. The spike is immediately inserted into the new bag (Figure 25E). A new connection shield is put around the spike/bag connection. The outlet port clamp is taken off. The new bag is hung up, the roller clamp is opened, and filling is started (Figure 25F). When filling is over, the roller clamp is closed and the empty bag is worn by the patient comfortably under the clothing (Figure 25G). The patient is allowed free activity while the solution is in the peritoneal cavity. At the end of the dwell time, the above-described exchanged procedure is repeated. Once every six months, a new transfer set is connected in place of the old one.

The basic Y-set procedure

The Y transfer set has a stem and two limbs, one for infusion and the other for drainage. At the time of exchange, a new full solution bag is connected to the infusion limb with the roller clamp in a closed position (Figure 26A) and an empty drain bag is attached to the drain limb (Figure 26B). The stem end is connected to the catheter end via a short straight transfer set (Figure 26C). The infusion and drainage limbs are flushed with a small amount of solution from the new bag (Figure 26D). Now the solution is drained from the peritoneal cavity into the empty drain bag (Figure 26E). The roller clamp on the drain limb is closed. The solution from the new bag is then infused into the peritoneal cavity. The Y transfer set is disconnected and discarded and the catheter end is capped (Figure 26F).

Bacteria that contaminate the transfer set at the time of connection with a new dialysis solution bag, are washed away into the drainage bag with a small volume of dialysis solution before the solution infusion into the peritoneal cavity is begun. This technique, called 'flush before fill' and introduced by Buoncristiani, minimizes the chances of bacterial contamination of the peritoneum and is the main advantage of the Y set (Figure 26 G–I).

The Y sets are available as either disposable single-use sets (A disconnect Y set with pre-attached 3-liter drain bag; Figure 23) or removable, reuse sets ('O' sets with an 8 week life), which incorporate flush-before-fill advantages of Y set systems and utilize an antiseptic which is stored in lines during dwell to disinfect the system.

Assist devices for CAPD

The assist devices, designed to reduce peritonitis, are portable, convenient, fast, and easy to use. Most of them have a lever-assisted exchange system that helps the patients, including those with visual and manual impairment, and easily connect the transfer set to the dialysis solution bags. In addition, some of these devices incorporate a sterilizing system that sterilizes the connection site before infusion.

Ultraviolet light devices

These devices have two components: (a) a mechanical system that conveniently assists the patients in spiking the transfer set to the dialysis solution bag, and (b) a UV light sterilization system that sterilizes the spike and port before they are connected.

Sterile connection device

This system welds the transfer set to the dialysis solution tubing with the help of a hot copper knife. The knife is heated to 260°C before it cuts through the tubing by melting. The heat of the knife sterilizes the cut ends as it cuts through.

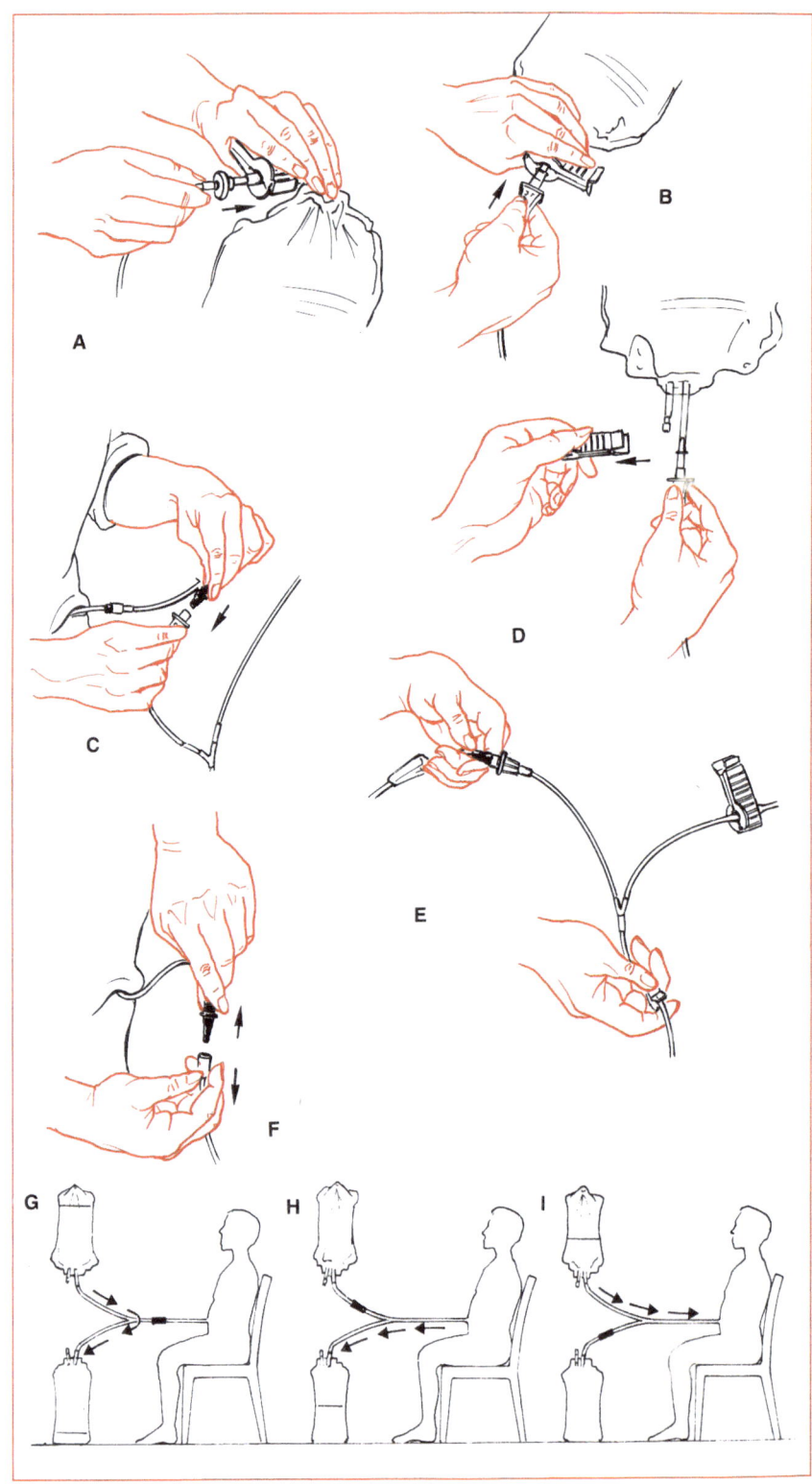

A

B

C

D

E

F

G   H   I

Peritoneal dialysis machines

The peritoneal dialysis machines (cyclers and proportioning units) are designed to deliver predetermined volumes of dialysis solution into the peritoneal cavity, and after a specified period of dwell time, drain it out. The cyclers use gravity for solution infusion and drainage, a heater for warming the solution to the body temperature, and valves to control the direction of solution flow to and from the peritoneal cavity. Some advanced cyclers incorporate electronic scales, drain alarms, and volume and time monitors. Proportioning units mix treated water with dialysis solution concentrate to produce large volumes of sterile solution and incorporate devices for solution inflow and outflow. These systems are no longer marketed due to low demand for the IPD therapy. A detailed description of cycler based peritoneal dialysis is given in Chapter 6 which deals with automated peritoneal dialysis.

◄─────────────────

Figure 26: The steps of basic Y set procedure
A *Attach drain bag*
B *Spike new solution bag*
C *Connect to set*
D *Flush*
E *Drain and infuse*
F *Disconnect*
G *Flush*
H *Drain*
I *Fill*

5 ACUTE PERITONEAL DIALYSIS

The main indications for acute peritoneal dialysis are (a) acute renal failure where recovery of renal function is anticipated, (b) initial dialysis in patients with end-stage renal disease, and (c) patients on chronic maintenance peritoneal dialysis hospitalized for intercurrent illness.

Access for acute peritoneal dialysis

Some centers use rigid catheters for peritoneal access in acute renal failure patients who require peritoneal dialysis for only a week or two. A semi-rigid plastic catheter comes with a metal stylet for piercing the abdominal wall (Figure 27). The steps of a rigid catheter insertion technique are described in Table 10 and Figures 28 and 29 show the rigid catheter in situ. Many centers prefer the insertion of a Tenckhoff catheter at the bedside

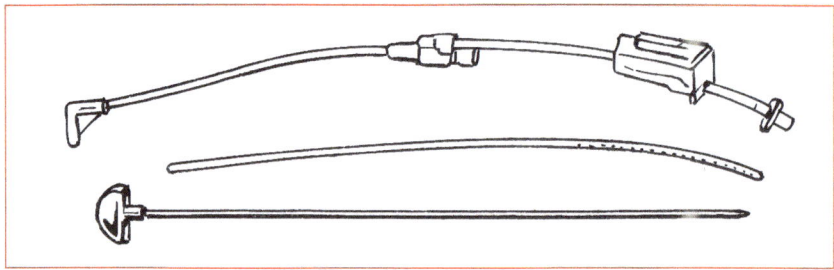

Figure 27: Illustrative diagram of a semi-rigid plastic catheter with its steel stylet and connecting tube.

TABLE 10.   Steps of a rigid catheter insertion technique in a patient with acute renal failure

1. Preparation of the patient should include cleaning the skin at the site of catheter in-
    sertion, emptying the bladder and bowel, an explanation of the procedure, and a pre-
    medication with a mild sedative (diazepam 5 mg orally or parenterally).
2. Sterile precaution should be followed including masking and gowning.
3. Choose the site of insertion (the best site for rigid is in the midline, 2–3 cm below the
    umbilicus) and anesthetize the skin with 2% xylocaine.
4. Through a small (2–3 mm) skin incision, a rigid catheter with the stylet in place is
    forced through the abdominal wall by a short thrust or rotating motion while the
    patient bears down firmly and distends the abdomen. While inserting, the catheter
    should be directed towards the coccyx for a pelvic placement. As the peritoneal
    cavity is entered, the loss of resistance is recognized as a 'pop'. At this time, the trocar
    is with-drawn slightly, and the catheter is advanced in the peritoneal cavity towards
    the pelvis. The pelvic placement is indicated by the patient as a pressure over the blad-
    der or rectum.
5. The catheter patency is checked with 2–3 solution exchanges. The catheter is secured
    to the skin with a metal disc (provided with the catheter) and tape (Figure 28).
6. A dry sterile dressing is applied over the incision. Figure 29 illustrates the position of a
    rigid catheter in relation to the internal organs in the peritoneal cavity.

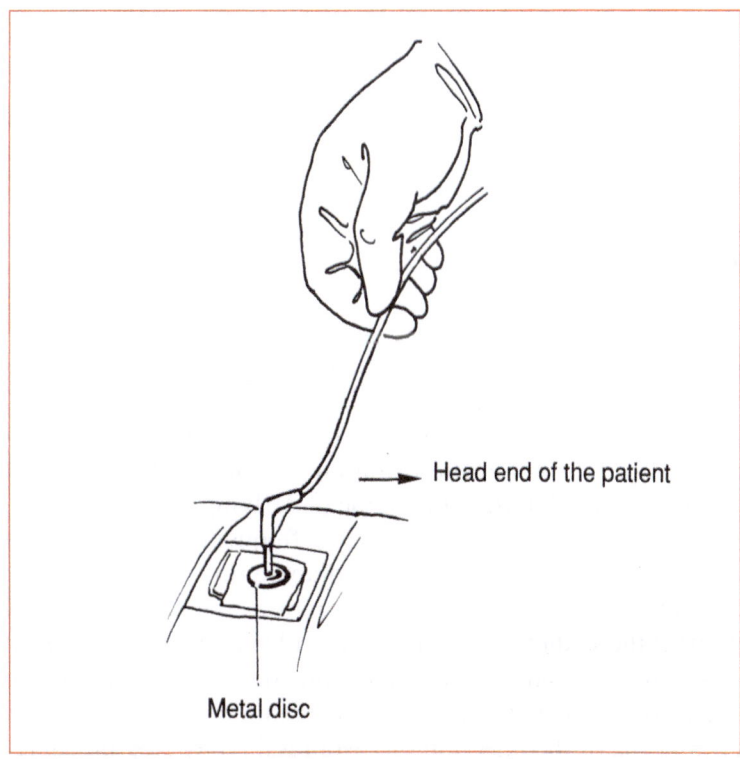

Head end of the patient

Metal disc

Figure 28: A rigid catheter attached to a connecting tube is fixed to the skin. A metal disc around the catheter stops the catheter from slipping into the peritoneal cavity.

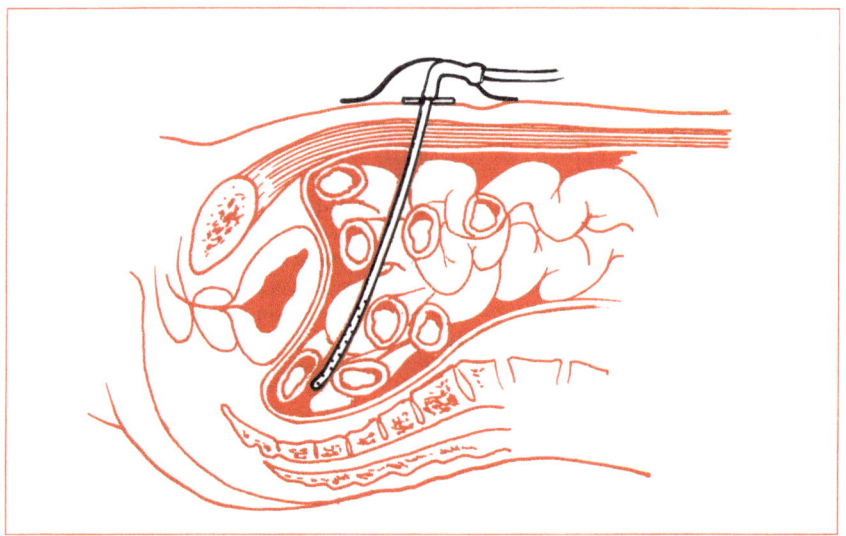

Figure 29: Illustration showing the position of a rigid catheter after insertion in relation to the abdominal wall and internal organs in the peritoneal cavity.

through a trocar or a guide wire. The steps of the trocar and guide wire insertion technique are detailed in Table 11.

Catheter complications

The rigid catheter insertion may be associated with several complications. About 7–10% of patients have inflow and outflow pain due to (a) pressure of the catheter tip on the internal organs, (b) acidic dialysis solution (pH 5.5), (c) hypertonic solution, (d) over-distension of the abdomen due to excessive fluid infusion or ultrafiltration, (e) entrapment of omentum in the catheter lumen. Identification of the underlying cause is crucial for relief of the pain. Shoulder or costal pain, a frequent occurrence, is usually due to an accumulation of air under the diaphragm.

Nearly half of the patients will have blood-stained exchanges immediately after the catheter insertion. This bleeding (usually minor) subsides after a few exchanges. Major bleeding may occur after traumatizing a large vessel or be due to uremic bleeding disorders. A transfusion of fresh blood or plasma or the injection of vasopressin may stop bleeding due to uremic bleeding disorders. Catheter blockage due to clots may be minimized by adding heparin in the dialysis solution.

TABLE 11.   Steps of insertion of a Tenckhoff catheter at the bedside (trocar and guide wire methods)

Trocar method:

1. The abdomen is shaved and the skin is cleaned.
2. The bladder and bowel are emptied.
3. A single dose of prophylactic antibiotic (Vancomycin 1 gm) is given.
4. Choose the site of insertion (preferred site for the bedside catheter insertion is in the midline, 2–3 cm below the umbilicus) and anesthetize the skin with 2% xylocaine.
5. A 2–3 cm midline incision is made and subcutaneous fat is dissected to the rectus sheath.
6. The peritoneal cavity may be filled with 1–2 liters of dialysis solution, especially in an unconscious patient.
7. A specially designed trocar (Figure 30) is introduced into the peritoneal cavity, while the patient bears down. While introducing, the trocar is directed towards the coccyx for a pelvic placement (Figure 31). As the peritoneal cavity is entered, the loss of resistance is recognized as a 'pop'. At this time, the central trocar is withdrawn, leaving the outer metal tube in place. A Tenckhoff catheter stiffened with a flexible metal rod is introduced into the peritoneal cavity through the metal tube and advanced to position it deep in the pelvic cavity. The flexible metal rod from the catheter is removed and the catheter is tested for patency by in-and-out saline or dialysis solution exchanges.
8. At this time the outer metal tube of the trocar is withdrawn. A purse string suture with an absorbable suture material is applied around the cuff, which is positioned close to the peritoneum.
9. The outer end of the catheter is brought out of the skin through a 2–3 inch subcutaneous tunnel. The skin incision closed with a running Mersilene suture. A sterile dress-

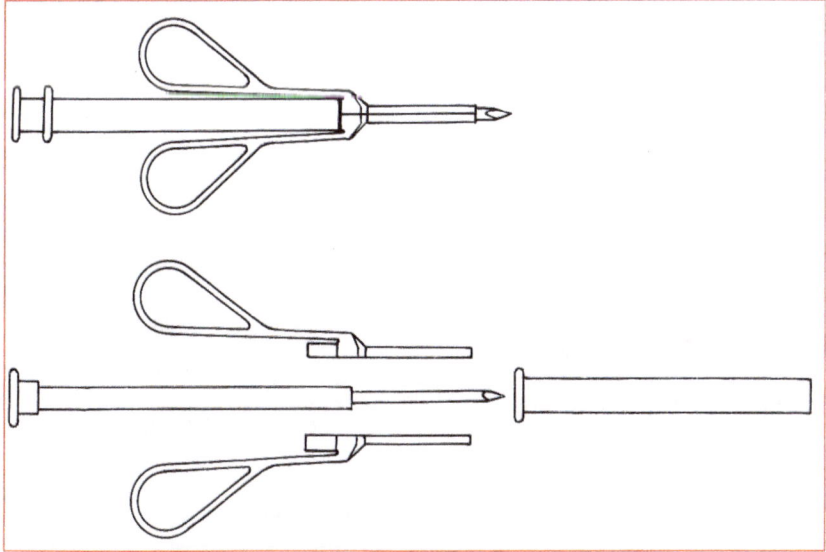

Figure 30: The Tenckhoff catheter introducer, fully assembled (above) and with parts separated (below).

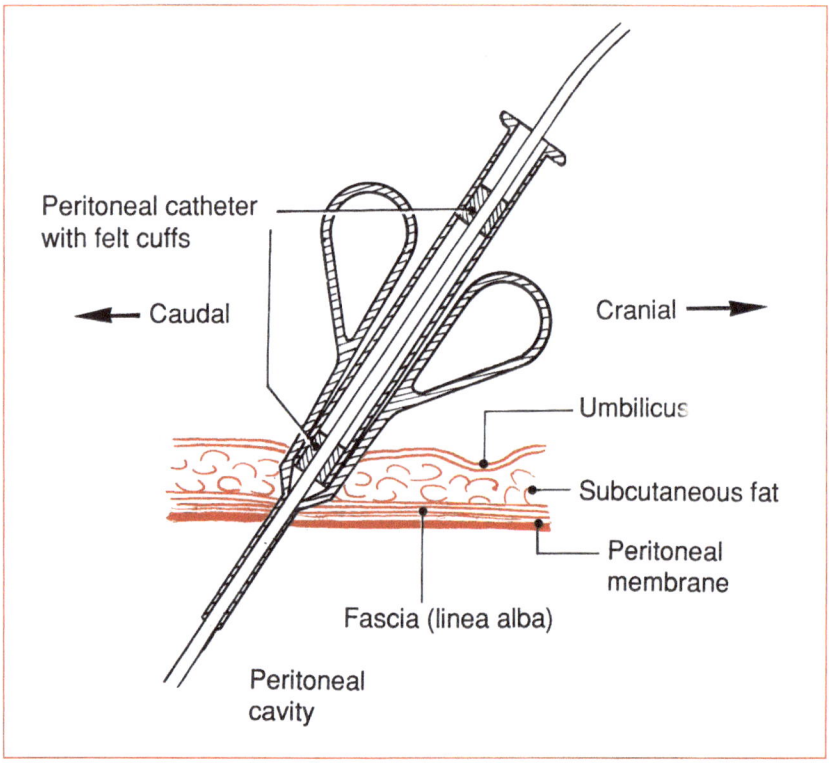

Figure 31: Illustration showing the position and direction of the trocar during the catheter insertion. Only the thin sharp tip of the fully assembled trocar penetrates the peritoneum. The thick tubular body is halted at the peritoneal level for positioning the internal cuff.

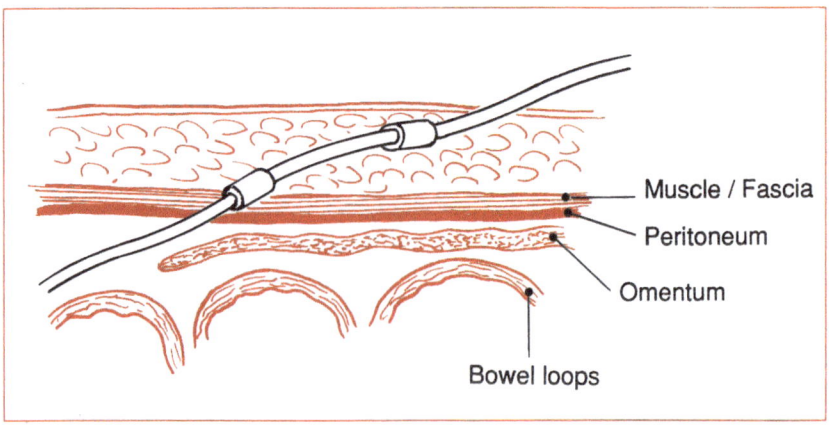

Figure 32: Illustration showing a peritoneal catheter in the abdominal wall with adjacent tissues.

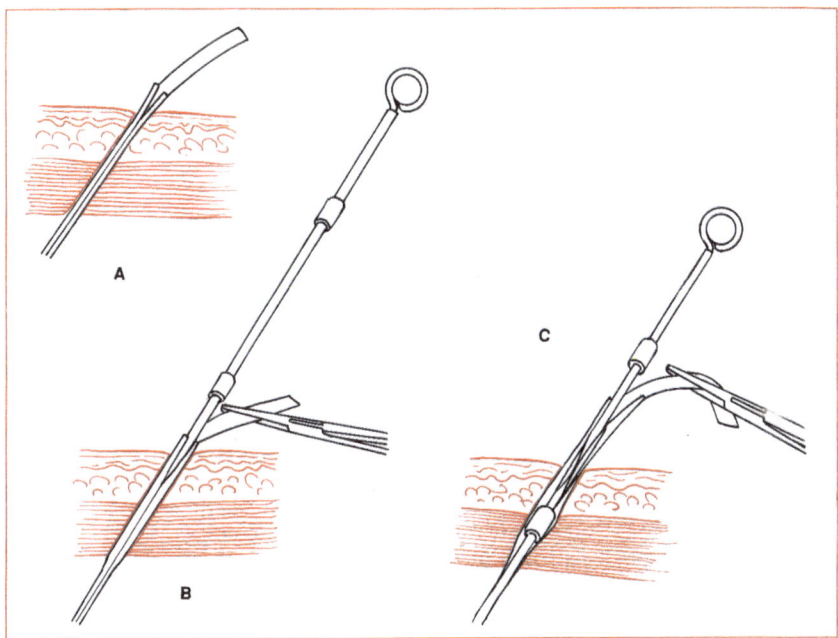

Figure 33 A–C: Steps of a guide wire insertion technique. (A): A stiff plastic tro-car surrounded by a thin pealable plastic Quill® in place in the abdominal wall, (B): a Tenckhoff catheter stiffened with a metal rod is introduced into the perito-neal cavity, (C): the outer thin plastic Quill® is pealed away. (Reproduced with permission from Medigroup, Inc., North Aurora, Illinois; Instructions on 'Perito-neoscopic placement of peritoneal dialysis catheters'.)

ing is applied around the incision. Figure 32 shows an illustrative diagram of a catheter in the abdominal wall with adjacent tissues.

10. A titanium adapter is connected to the outer end of the catheter and dialysis exchanges are resumed.

Guide wire technique:

1. The initial steps are similar to steps 1–6 of the trocar insertion technique.
2. Insert the guide wire into the peritoneal cavity through the needle used for fluid infu-sion. The needle is removed, leaving the guide wire in place.
3. A dilator, covered in a perforated sheath is inserted into the peritoneal cavity by ad-vancing it around the guide wire. Now the guide wire and dilator are withdrawn, leaving the sheath in place
4. A Tenckhoff catheter stiffened with a flexible metal rod is introduced into the perito-neal cavity through the plastic sheath and advanced to position the catheter tip in the pelvic cavity. The flexible metal rod from the catheter is removed and the catheter is tested for patency by 2–3 dialysis solution exchanges. At this time, the outer thin sheath is withdrawn by peeling. A purse-string suture with an absorbable suture material is applied around the cuff which is positioned close to the peritoneum.
5. The final steps are similar to steps 9 and 10 of the trocar technique.

Dialysis solution leakage is the most troublesome complication of catheter insertion. The risk of leakage increases with frequent catheter manipulations, especially in patients with lax abdominal walls. Excessive fluid infusion may also cause fluid leakage. The dialysis fluid may extravasate into the abdominal wall if the rigid catheter is inadvertently inserted into the potential space between the layers of abdominal wall.

Poor drainage may be due to any one of the following causes: (a) fibrin or a clot blocking the terminal holes of the catheter, (b) pressure on the catheter from internal organs, (c) preperitoneal placement of the catheter, and (d) intra-abdominal adhesions. The first condition benefits from catheter irrigation. Repositioning or reinsertion of the catheter may be necessary for all of the other causes.

Organ perforation is rare, but may occur occasionally in susceptible patients. The conditions that increase the risk of perforation are paralytic ileus, bowel obstruction, unconsciousness or heavy sedation, and previous severe acute intra-abdominal sepsis with adhesions. Clinical evidence of acute perforation are: sudden sharp or severe abdominal pain followed by watery diarrhea, poor solution outflow, and cloudy, foul-smelling effluent mixed with fecal material, etc. The perforation usually completely seals off within 24 hours after removal of the catheter but surgical intervention may be necessary if the perforation is large, especially in the colon.

Prolonged use of a rigid catheter is associated with a high incidence of peritonitis. The treatment of peritonitis is described in detail elsewhere.

Prescription of acute peritoneal dialysis

The acute peritoneal dialysis prescription, which specifies the duration of each dialysis session, the exchange volume and period, the dialysis solution flow rate, glucose concentration and additives, and the method of exchange (manual or cycler), is tailored to the individual patient's needs.

The duration of each treatment could vary from 24 to 72 hours depending on the severity of uremia. Because of the slower solute removal compared to a hemodialysis treatment, prolonged peritoneal dialysis therapy seldom causes a disequilibrium syndrome. The dialysis solution volume of each exchange is dictated by the size and age of the patients. An average adult patient can easily tolerate a 2-liter volume without much discomfort. Patients with smaller body size, recent abdominal incisions, and hernias are best managed with lower exchange volumes. A dialysis solution flow

TABLE 12. Composition of bicarbonate peritoneal dialysis solution, prepared in the hospital pharmacy

	Amount added
$NaHCO_3$ (7.5%)	80 ml
5% Dextrose	667 ml
NaCl (0.9%)	1333 ml

This mixture will contain	Concentration
Bicarbonate	34.4 mEq/liter
Sodium	133 mEq/liter
Chloride	98.5 mEq/liter
Dextrose	160 g/liter
Calcium / magnesium	0

rate of 2–3 liter/hr provides the most cost-effective dialysis. During an exchange, inflow and outflow times are kept as low (4–5 minutes per liter for inflow and 5–10 minutes per liter for outflow) as possible. Choice of dialysis solution dextrose concentration is guided by the amount of ultrafiltration needed.

In patients with an average peritoneal solute transport rate, a 2-liter 1.5% dextrose solution over a 60 minute dwell typically yields about 50–100 ml of ultrafiltration volume. Higher dextrose concentrations (2.5% = 100–200, and 4.25% = 300–400 ml) would provide proportionally higher ultrafiltration. During an acute episode of peritonitis, the peritoneal membrane becomes hyperpermeable and permits rapid dissipation of the glucose gradient, resulting in lower net ultrafiltration.

TABLE 13. Complications of acute peritoneal dialysis

Catheter complications
        inflow and outflow pain
        blood stained exchanges
        dialysis solution leak
        poor drainage
        perforation or laceration of organs
        Vaso-vagal attack
Medical complications
        peritonitis
        hyper and hypovolemia
        arrhythmia
        hyper and hypoglycemia
        hypernatremia
        hypokalemia
        atelectasis
        aspiration pneumonia

If rigid catheters are used for access, a prophylactic intraperitoneal antibiotic (cephalothin (100 mg/liter) for reducing the risk of infection, and heparin (500 units/liter) to prevent blockage of the catheter), may be necessary for the first 24 to 36 hours. A potassium-free dialysis solution is employed in peritoneal dialysis for most renal failure patients because the peritoneal membrane clears potassium slowly, and these patients have a tendency toward hyperkalemia. However, if a patient is receiving digoxin, especially during the initial dialysis, potassium should be added to the dialysis solution (2-4 mEq/liter) to avoid sudden changes in serum potassium and prevent myocardial irritability and potential fatal arrhythmia.

Occasionally, patients unable to metabolize lactate (e.g., those in hepatic failure or with severe lactic acidosis) may need a dialysis solution containing bicarbonate. Table 12 shows the composition of this solution which, if used for more than 24 hours, may induce serious calcium and magnesium losses. Hence, these ions should be replaced intravenously. On the other hand, this type of dialysis solution may be used for the treatment of hypercalcemia.

A peritoneal dialysis treatment for acute renal failure should typically last for 48 to 72 hours. It is important that the dialysis orders for the acute treatment be written for 24 hours only. At the end of each 24 hours, the patient should be reassessed and modified orders should be written if necessary. Acutely sick patients with unstable vital signs will need more frequent re-evaluation.

The complications encountered during an acute peritoneal dialysis are listed in Table 13. A well functioning catheter is a must for a trouble-free dialysis. The medical complications are usually a result of rapid alteration of hemodynamic status brought about by the dialysis. A careful and planned removal of fluid avoids hyper or hypovolemia. Tachyarrhythmias are frequent in patients with known cardiac disease. A rapid fluid shift may be deleterious to such patients. Prolonged dialysis of over 48 to 72 hours in a supine position may predispose an acutely sick patient to hypoxia, basal atelectasis, and aspiration pneumonia.

It is necessary to monitor the blood sugar closely in patients, especially diabetics, for hyperglycemia when frequent hypertonic dextrose solutions are used. Diabetic patients will require insulin over and above their daily requirement. Insulin could be given either subcutaneously or intraperitoneally. When given intraperitoneally, insulin is omitted from the last 2–4 exchanges mainly to avoid hypoglycemia.

Mild degrees of hypernatremia are common following ultrafiltration using hypertonic glucose solutions. At those times, more water than sodium is lost from the vascular compartment due to sodium sieving. To prevent severe degrees of hypernatremia, it is recommended to replace one-half of the net ultrafiltration with water intravenously or by mouth, or by the use of a solution with a sodium concentration calculated to yield a sieving coefficient near 1. Substitution of 5% glucose and water for every sixth or eighth liter of dialysate may also prevent hypernatremia.

Patients on acute peritoneal dialysis may develop either respiratory or metabolic alkalosis. The former may develop during the initial stages of dialysis when hyperventilation, due to a low spinal fluid pH, may continue to reduce P_{CO_2}, while serum bicarbonate increases as the body generates bicarbonate to correct the extracellular acidosis. Since the bicarbonate ions diffuse slowly across the blood-brain barrier, cerebrospinal fluid pH does not change promptly and the respiratory center continues to drive hyperventilation, further reducing P_{CO_2}. This tendency may be slight during dialysis because lactate conversion to bicarbonate in the liver occurs slowly enough to permit the CSF pH to adjust. In view of this cycle of events, one should not infuse bicarbonate to achieve rapid correction of acidosis. Uremic patients, who also have liver failure may have difficulty in converting lactate to bicarbonate and, as a result, the blood lactate rises. This problem may be corrected by the parenteral infusion of bicarbonate or by the use of bicarbonate instead of lactate in the blood.

6 AUTOMATED PERITONEAL DIALYSIS

Over the past five years, compared to CAPD, there has been a rapid growth of automated peritoneal dialysis (APD). In APD therapy, a cycler machine is used for infusion and drainage of the dialysis solution (Figure 34). The growth of APD has resulted from a combination of improved physician knowledge of the peritoneal physiology and the availability of better cycler machines for patient use. The physicians have learned to prescribe an adequate amount of dialysis by using adequacy measures such as the dialysis creatinine clearance and Kt/V urea, etc. CAPD patients, either inadequately dialyzed because of the low peritoneal membrane function or unable to continue on CAPD because of the complications resulting from raised intra-abdominal pressure, who otherwise would have dropped out from the peritoneal dialysis treatment, are being increasingly managed by the APD therapy.

The assessment of peritoneal equilibration rates of patients has allowed the identification of unsuitable patients for long-term CAPD and the institution of APD prescription in a timely manner. Recently, more versatile cycler machines have been introduced which enable physicians to tailor the dialysis prescription to the patient's needs. The current cyclers are capable of delivering varying amounts of solution volumes (minimum volume of 50 ml) with increments of 10 ml per exchange. This cycler capability has allowed pediatric patients to use APD extensively for chronic dialysis treatment. Some of the newer cyclers are devised to exchange solutions based on a predetermined fixed drain volume rather than a dwell time. This cycler potential has allowed patients to carry out tidal peritoneal dialysis (TPD). During a TPD session, a large volume of solution (up to 30 liters) is exchanged in a short time (8–10 hours) through the fast cycling technique. By allowing a reserve volume of solution into the perito-

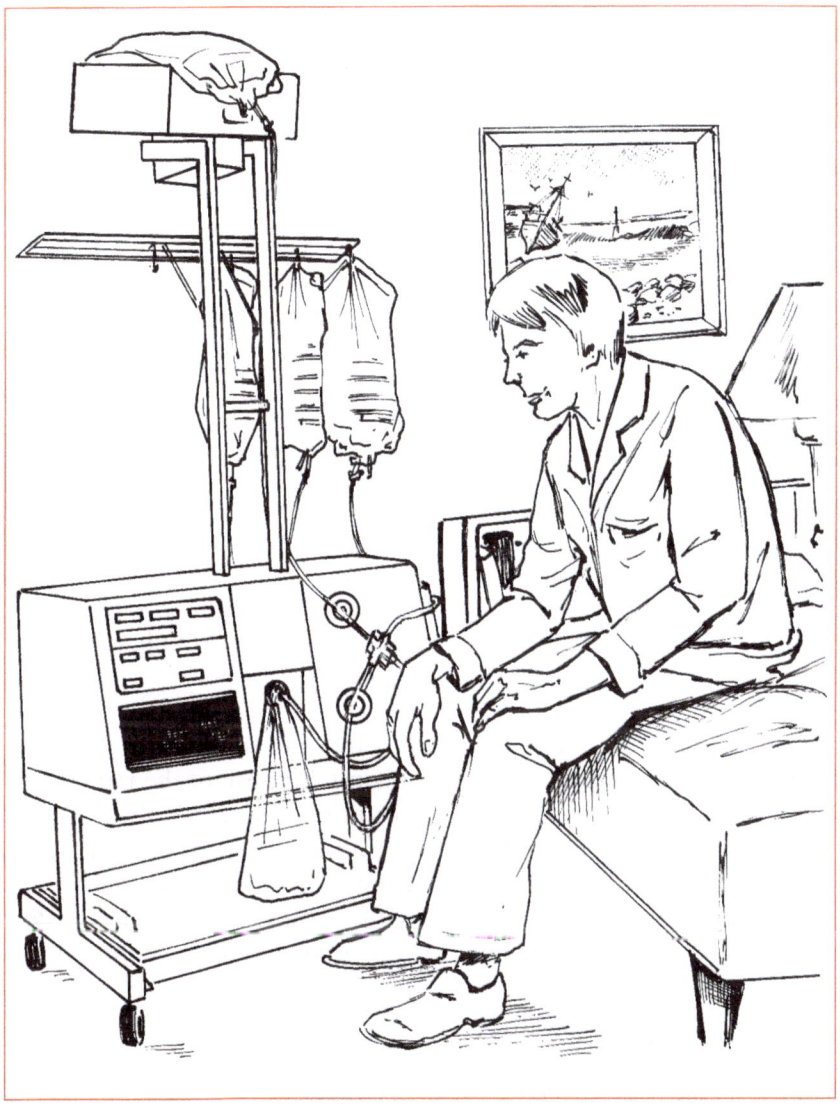

Figure 34: Patient on Automated Peritoneal Dialysis with cycler machine used for infusion and drainage of the dialysis solution.

neal cavity throughout the treatment session, the dead exchange time (the time during infusion and drainage when the dialysis solution is incapable of sufficient membrane contact) is minimized. By using the TPD technique, the efficiency of peritoneal dialysis can be improved by about 20% compared to IPD using a similar volume of dialysis solution. The newer cyclers are safer and capable of monitoring multiple parameters of dialysis indices such as infusion, drainage and ultrafiltration volumes.

TABLE 14.   The peritoneal dialysis regimens that utilize a cycler machine for infusion and drainage of dialysis solution

Daily (night or day) intermittent peritoneal dialysis (NIPD)
    (a) last bag option during the day,
    (b) dry day.
Intermittent peritoneal dialysis (two to three weekly sessions)
Continuous cyclic peritoneal dialysis (CCPD)
    (a) last bag option during the day,
    (b) dry day.
Tidal peritoneal dialysis (TPD)
    (a) last bag option during the day,
    (b) dry day.

The peritoneal dialysis regimens that utilize the cyclers for the APD therapy, either totally or part of the time, are listed in Table 14. The indications for APD are listed in Table 15.

> The patient who is estimated to have a high solute equilibration rate on peritoneal equilibration test is best suited for APD because of the ability to provide short exchange dialysis.

Since the peak ultrafiltration volume is achieved early in an exchange in a patient with a high equilibration rate mainly because of the rapid loss of glucose gradient due to brisk glucose absorption from the solution, a short exchange allows for the capture of ultrafiltration at its peak. The cycler permits multiple short exchanges during a session of treatment which could conveniently be performed during the night when the patient is sleeping and allows the daytime for normal function without the burden of hav-

TABLE 15.   Indications for APD

1. Personal patient preference.
2. Specific peritoneal membrane characteristic.
    (a) high solute equilibration rate to provide short exchange dialysis,
    (b) low average equilibration rate to provide high dose and/or high volume dialysis.
3. Pre-existing medical conditions which could become aggravated due to increased intra-abdominal pressure, i.e. hernia, COPD, etc.
4. Malnourished patients who require parenteral nutrition, to achieve higher ultrafiltration.
5. Pediatric or geriatric patients who require a partner to conduct dialysis.
6. Special job requirement that may not permit or be conducive to perform CAPD at work.

ing to perform sterile dialysis exchanges. The timing of a cycler session is best left to the patient's convenience. The APD patients who cannot be adequately dialyzed during the time period that is convenient and practical (8–10 hours a day), have the option of using additional daytime exchanges to provide incremental dialysis clearance.

A patient with a high peritoneal solute equilibration rate is best suited for the IPD therapy. Because of the faster rate of solute transfer, adequate clearance for small solutes can be achieved in a shorter time period. However, APD therapy may be inadequate for clearance of large solutes, which need longer treatment time. Adequate dialysis can be provided to patients with low average solute equilibration rates, by the high dose and high volume APD treatment. For up to one to two years after initiating dialysis, the contribution of the residual renal function to overall solute clearance can be significant, particularly for patients with low average or low peritoneal solute equilibration rates. It is important to emphasize the fact that these patients can develop subtle signs of uremia with the gradual loss of residual renal function with time. In many of these patients, especially those with a large body mass, the APD treatment alone might be insufficient to provide adequate dialysis, in which case serious consideration should be given for switching the patients to hemodialysis.

The main advantage of APD is its flexibility. The treatment sessions can be adjusted to the patient's convenience. Dialysis prescription can be tailored to the patient's convenience and peritoneal function characteristics. Compared to CAPD, the number of connection/disconnections are fewer during APD, especially with CCPD, and this has resulted in lower rates of peritonitis in experienced centers.

Clinical experiences with APD therapy have indicated that outcome measures of dialysis are comparable to CAPD therapy. The uremic complications such as anemia, pericarditis, neuropathy, and osteodystrophy are controlled just as well as on CAPD therapy. The nutritional status of patients receiving adequate APD is comparable to CAPD patient. Blood pressure control during APD may not be as good as CAPD due to lower sodium removal (sodium sieving) during rapid ultrafiltration. Nevertheless, sufficient sodium could be removed during a treatment session to maintain a good sodium balance and blood pressure control.

The peritoneal equilibration test is helpful in many ways for APD therapy. An individual patient's peritoneal membrane solute equilibration rate is important in determining the bag option during the day. A patient with a high solute equilibration rate may retain fluid during a long dwell exchange, whereas another patient with a low equilibration rate may find him or herself underdialyzed if dialysis exchanges are done only during the limited hours of night. If the total amount of creatinine clearance to be given is known, and the predicted D/P ratio of creatinine for a given dwell time is determined from PET curve, then the total duration of an APD session can be determined by

$$T_d = \frac{K_d \times 168}{K_{di}},$$

where K_d is the total amount of average weekly dialysis creatinine clearance (ml/min) to be provided (targeted value), K_{di} is the APD therapy creatinine clearance (ml/min) determined from the PET curve (D/P × drainage volume per exchange), T_d is the therapy time in hours/week, and 168 is the number of hours in a week. Conversely, if the total clearance and duration of a session is known, the duration of an exchange can be determined.

Good catheter function is essential for successful APD therapy. A poorly functioning catheter will cause frequent alarms during the treatment time. Also, drainage time will be prolonged (> 20 min for a 2-liter volume) and contributes to loss of dialysis time.

Blood-sugar control of diabetic patients on APD treatment is achieved by giving insulin in the following way:

(a) Control of blood sugar using SC insulin during the day as per standard practice of blood-sugar control.
(b) During the night when the cycler is used to cover for the dialysis-associated glucose load, insulin may be given in one of the following ways
    (i) SC long-acting insulin (dose varies from patient to patient). Potential for hypoglycemia exists if dialysis is prematurely terminated for any reason;
    (ii) intraperitoneal regular insulin through the bags (amount of insulin needed should be individualized).

The main limitation of the APD therapy at present is the inability to provide adequate dialysis in a time span that is practical, i.e. 8–9 hours a session, especially for the patients with a less-than-average transport function, and the higher cost compared to standard CAPD / CCPD.

7 ADEQUACY OF DIALYSIS

Clinical indicators

The primary goal of dialysis is to maintain a uremic patient in the best possible physical condition and to prevent complications due to uremic toxicity, by providing as much dialysis as practically possible and economically feasible. Clinical and laboratory indicators of an adequately dialyzed patient are shown in Table 16.

Blood urea nitrogen alone is a poor indicator of dialysis adequacy because its level is significantly influenced by the dietary protein intake.

TABLE 16. Clinical and laboratory indices of adequate peritoneal dialysis

Clinical
   Patient feels well.
   Blood pressure well controlled.
   Stable lean body mass.
   Good fluid balance.
   Absence of uremic symptoms such as anorexia, loss of appetite, loss of taste, insomnia, asthenia, etc.

Laboratory
   Serum creatinine <16–20 mg/dl (muscular person) or <12–15 mg/dl (thin and lean person).
   Normal serum electrolytes including calcium, phosphorus, and magnesium.
   Stable nerve conduction velocities.
   Normal serum albumin.

Adequacy indices

The amount of dialysis given to a patient can be determined by either normalized creatinine clearance (usually per 1.73 m^2 BSA) or normalized urea clearance (usually per total body water, V; K_t / V). Dietary protein intake (DI) can be estimated from the protein catabolic rate (PCR), which can be calculated from urea kinetics.

Creatinine clearance (C_{cr}) measurements

Net mean peritoneal clearance is determined for a continuous treatment (CAPD or CCPD) by dividing the amount of creatinine removed through dialysis per unit time (mass transfer rate) by the concentration of creatinine in the serum:

$$C_{cr} = \frac{(D_t \times V_t) - (D_o \times V_o)}{P},$$

where D_t and D_o are the final and infused dialysis solution creatinine concentrations, V_t and V_o are the final and initial dialysis solution volumes, and P is the serum creatinine concentration.

Since the infused solution is devoid of creatinine, the equation can be simplified to:

$$C_{cr} = \frac{(D_t \times V_t)}{P}.$$

This clearance expresses the volume of serum cleared of creatinine per unit time (usually expressed as milliliters per minute) by the peritoneal membrane. Clearance is influenced by dialysis flow rate, ultrafiltration, and membrane area and permeability, and is independent of blood concentration. The mean net clearance rate may be calculated per exchange, per day, or per week. The true instantaneous clearance rate is highest at the beginning of dialysis and approaches zero at equilibrium.

Residual renal function contributes to the overall clearance of small and middle molecular weight solutes and fluid removal. In some CAPD patients, significant residual renal function may help lessen the number and/or volume of exchanges. Since the renal creatinine clearance overestimates the glomerular filtration rate (GFR) in chronic renal failure patients, the average of renal creatinine and urea clearance may be added to the peritoneal creatinine clearance to estimate the combined or dialysis and GFR clearance provided to a patient on peritoneal dialysis.

Past experiences with peritoneal dialysis patients have indicated that patients do well when they receive dialysis which along with GFR provides a creatinine clearance of at least 5 ml/min (50 liter/week). The morbidity and mortality of such patients are lower compared to patients receiving lower amounts of clearance.

Based on clinical experiences, it is recommended that, to remain symptom free, anuric patients on CAPD/CCPD should receive dialysis which provides a combined creatinine clearance (peritoneal + residual renal GFR) of at least 50 liter/week/1.73 m^2 body surface area. Patients receiving dialysis with creatinine clearance values between 40 and 50 liter/week/1.73 m^2 need close observation for signs of inadequate dialysis.

With intermittent dialysis therapy, average weekly dialysis creatinine clearance is calculated based on the formula

$$K_d = \frac{K_{di} \times T_d}{168},$$

where K_d is the minimum required average weekly dialysis creatinine clearance (ml/min), K_{di} is the intermittent therapy creatinine clearance (ml/min), T_d is the therapy time in hours/week, and 168 is the number of hours in a week. If the minimum required dialysis creatinine clearance (K_d) is 5.5 ml/min and the patient's intermittent therapy creatinine clearance (K_{di}) is 12 ml/min (calculated during the therapy for at least three exchanges), the minimum required dialysis time per week can be calculated by:

$$T_d = \frac{K_d \times 168}{K_{di}}$$

or

$$T_d = \frac{5.5 \times 168}{12} = 77 \text{ hours/week.}$$

The steps of measuring combined creatinine clearance for a continuous treatment such as CAPD or CCPD are shown in Table 17 and for intermittent treatment are shown in Table 18.

TABLE 17. Steps for calculating the combined creatinine clearance (renal + peritoneal) for patients on CAPD

(A) Collect and measure the 24 hours volumes of dialysate and urine; take a sample from the dialysate and urine and measure the creatinine concentrations.
(B) Determine the serum creatinine concentration on the day of volume collection.
(C) Calculate the peritoneal creatinine clearance

$$C_p \text{ (liter/day)} = \frac{D_t \times V_t}{P},$$

where C_p is the peritoneal creatinine clearance, D_t is the dialysis solution creatinine concentration, V_t is the dialysis solution volume, and P is the serum creatinine concentration.
(D) Calculate the residual renal creatinine and urea clearances

$$C_R \text{ (liter/day)} = \frac{U \times V}{P},$$

where C_R is the renal urea or creatinine clearance, U is the urine urea nitrogen or creatinine concentration (mg/liter), and P is the serum urea nitrogen or creatinine (mg/liter). Calculate the mean of C_{urea} and C_{cr} to gel the 'average' clearance, which is a close estimation of GFR
(E) Combined creatinine clearance:

$$\text{liter/day} = C_p + C_R,$$

$$\text{ml/min} = \frac{(C_p + C_R) \times 1000}{1440}.$$

In patients with low peritoneal equilibration rates, the solute equilibration increases almost linearly during an exchange. Consequently, clearance per exchange increases almost linearly throughout the long exchange. For such patients, total dialysis time is critical for adequate clearance and continuous regimens such as CAPD or CCPD should be preferred over intermittent regimens.

In patients with high peritoneal transport rates, dialysate to plasma ratios of small solutes approach unity by 4 hours. By this time, the intraperitoneal volume is decreasing due to absorption. Therefore, clearances beyond 4 hours decrease proportionately. Reducing the dwell time in these patients captures better ultrafiltration than long dwell exchanges, while maintaining solute equilibration near unity; consequently, clearances are also higher. These patients therefore benefit more from rapid exchange techniques utilizing a cycler such as NIPD, NTPD, IPD, etc.

TABLE 18. Steps for calculating the combined peritoneal and renal clearance for patients on IPD/NIPD/TPD

(A) Collect and measure the volume of dialysate during a dialysis session; take a sample of dialysate and measure the creatinine concentration.
(B) Estimate the serum creatinine pre- and post-dialysis and calculate the average of the two values.
(C) Collect and measure the volume of urine during a 24 hours period of dialysis; take a sample and measure the creatinine concentration.
(D) Estimate the serum creatinine pre- and post-urine collection and calculate the average of the two values.
(E) Calculate the peritoneal creatinine clearance.

$$C_p \text{ (liter/day)} = \frac{D_t \times V_t}{P_a},$$

where P_a is the average of pre- and post- serum creatine concentrations.
(F) Calculate the renal creatinine clearance

$$C_R \text{ (liter/day)} = \frac{U \times V}{P_a},$$

calculate the renal C_{urea} similary and average C_{urea} and C_{cr} to gel the 'average' C_{cr} by GFR.
(G) Calculate the combined creatinine clearance per day:
Combined creatinine clearance

(liter/day) $= C_p + C_R$,
(liter/week) $= (C_p + C_R) \times 7$

(H) Calculate IPD clearance:

$$C_{IPD} \text{(liter/day)} = \frac{D_t \times V_t}{P_a \times t},$$

Patients with high-average solute transport rates can be easily managed with many PD regimens. Figure 18 depicts the algorithm providing choices of PD therapy based on peritoneal solute transport rates measured by the peritoneal equilibration test.

Urea kinetic parameters

Until recently, urea kinetics were used for assessing the adequacy of small solute removal, mainly in hemodialysis. Gotch and Sargent introduced the term Kt/V as an index of hemodialysis adequacy, where K is the urea clearance, t the treatment time, and V the volume of urea distribution in the

TABLE 19.   Steps for calculating Kt/V and protein catabolic rate (PRC) for CAPD patients

(A) Calculate the combined peritoneal and renal urea clearance as per Table 17.
(B) Since CAPD is a continuous treatment, the combined dialysis and renal urea clearance per day represents the term Kt.
(C) Estimate the volume of urea distribution in the body water by Watson nomogram, which takes into account sex, age, height, and weight (lean body mass).
(D) Calculate the Kt/V (urea clearance/volume of urea distribution).
(E) Calculate PCR (gm/day) = 10.76 (G_u + 1.46), where G_u = urea generation rate (mg/min) (G_u = the mg of urea in the 24 hour (urine + dialysate)/1440).

total body water. The term expresses the urea clearance normalized for its volume of distribution in the total body water. The morbidity and mortality of hemodialysis patients are lower when they receive dialysis which provides a Kt/V of at least 1 per treatment or 3 per week compared to those with a Kt/V of 0.6 or 1.8 per week.

Similarly, the importance of protein intake to the adequacy of dialysis is reflected by the observation that a protein catabolic rate (PCR) below 0.8 gm/kg normalized body weight/day is associated with a high morbidity in hemodialysis patients. Several studies have shown a close correlation between the PCR and dietary protein intake (DPI) calculated from dietetic history. Well-dialyzed hemodialysis patients eat well and have a good nutritional status and have a PCR of 1 or above. Their serum albumin is in the normal range. Serum albumin is a good predictor of long-term survival in dialysis patients.

Recently, Keshaviah and Nolph have applied the Kt/V method of adequacy measurement to CAPD patients. Preliminary observations indicate that, for adequate dialysis, CAPD patients require a Kt/V of 1.7/week or more and patients with a Kt/V of 1.4/week or less present clinical evidence of inadequate dialysis. Well-dialyzed CAPD patients often have a PCR of at least 0.9 gm/kg ($V/0.58$). The details of calculating Kt/V for CAPD patients are given in Table 19.

Preliminary indications suggest that weekly Kt/V levels of 1.9 for CAPD patients are equivalent to a hemodialysis Kt/V of 3 per week or 1 per treatment. Kt/V levels between 1.4 to 1.7 are considered marginal and such patients need close observations for signs of inadequate dialysis. In CAPD patients who have a weekly Kt/V of over 1.7, PCR has been reported to be about 0.9 gm/kg ($V/0.58$)/day.

It is important to recognize the relationship between the weekly creatinine clearance and weekly Kt/V urea, especially in patients who are transferred from a long-cycle therapy, such as CAPD, to a short-cycle technique, such as NIPD. With a long-cycle therapy, the ratio of weekly creatinine clearance to weekly Kt/V urea is higher than with a short cycle therapy in the same patient. If patients are shifted from CAPD to NIPD and maintain the same weekly creatinine clearance, then the weekly Kt/V urea will increase.

Mass transfer area coefficient

This coefficient represents the clearance rate that would be realized in the absence of both ultrafiltration and solute accumulation in the dialysate. The calculation is based on kinetic models and incorporates several assumptions as to the movement of solutes between body compartments, contributions of convective transport, absence of blood flow limitation on solute movement, and amplification relative to inflow and drainage. This index is primarily a research tool and is seldom used in clinical practice because of the complex calculations required for its determination.

Several other adequacy indices (dialysis index, drain volume index) have been proposed for measuring the adequacy of peritoneal dialysis. These indices are based on clearance measurements or drain volumes and, thus, have no additional benefits over clearance or Kt/V indices.

8 PERITONITIS AND EXIT-SITE INFECTION

Peritonitis had been recognized as the most frequent and potentially therapy-limiting complication of CAPD. In the early years of CAPD, it accounted for nearly 50% of hospitalizations in CAPD patients.

In recent years, a dramatic reduction in the incidence of peritonitis has occurred, mainly due to improved techniques and connector technology. The incidence reported with the use of Y-set connectors has ranged from one episode every two to three years.

Peritonitis during chronic intermittent therapy, where the number of connect/disconnects per session are fewer and are performed by nurses, is lower than that in CAPD patients.

Most peritonitis episodes in CAPD patients (about 75%) are due to organisms which are normal skin and nasal flora, i.e., *Staphylococcus aureus* and *epidermidis*. The route of entry and the common organisms causing peritonitis are listed in Table 20.

External contamination of the dialysis delivery system, mainly at the connection site of the transfer set and the bag during the exchange procedure, is probably the foremost source of bacterial entry into the peritoneal cavity.

Infrequently water borne organisms such as *Acinetobacter*, and *Pseudomonas* sp. may contaminate the connection site and be responsible for peritonitis. Another common source of bacteria causing peritonitis may be along the exterior surface of the indwelling catheter via the exit site and tunnel. The common organisms that infect the exit site and tunnel are

TABLE 20. Routes of infection and the common type of organisms causing peritonitis during CAPD

Route	Organisms
(A) Contamination at connection sites	*Staphylococcus epidermidis, Staphylococcus aureus, Acinetobacter*
(B) Pericatheter (exit site or tunnel infection)	*Staph epi, Staph aureus, Pseudomonas, Proteus,* yeast
(C) Transmural (through the gut wall)	Multiple organisms in association with anaerobes and fungi
(D) Hemotogenous	*Streptococcus, Mycrobacterium*
(E) Ascending (through the vagina)	*Pseudomonas,* yeast

Staphylococcus aureus and *epidermidis, Diphtheroides,* and a host of gram negative organisms, such as *Pseudomonas* and *Proteus,* etc. Transmural migration of micro-organisms from the gut lumen to the peritoneal cavity can cause peritonitis usually in association with internal inflammation such as diverticulitis, appendicitis, cholecystitis, etc. Commonly, peritonitis from a visceral leak is due to organisms belonging to more than one species and frequently dialysate contains anaerobic organisms or fungi. Hematogenous and other endogenous infections cause peritonitis infrequently.

A peritonitis episode due to *S. epidermidis* is usually mild and resolves quickly with appropriate antibiotic treatment. In contrast, peritonitis due to *S. aureus* has a much more severe and prolonged course, with a tendency for abscess formation. Occasional patients may be in severe shock at the initial presentation. *S. aureus* peritonitis usually responds well to appropriate antibiotic treatment, but the response is slower than that of *S. epidermidis* peritonitis. Because of the tendency of *Staphylococci* to survive in intracellular form, recurrences are frequent with both *S. epidermidis* and *aureus* infections. Treatment with a combination of a penicillin-type antibiotic and rifampin is useful for the prevention of recurrence. If infection is found in association with catheter exit-site infection from the same organism, catheter removal becomes necessary for cure. *Streptococcus viridans* causes severe peritonitis with marked constitutional symptoms but easily responds to treatment. Anaerobic infections usually indicate a bowel perforation, have a high propensity for abscess formation, and require aggressive surgical management.

Pseudomonas infections are a potentially serious problem. They are usually refractory to antibiotic treatment and often cause abscesses in the peritoneal cavity. Most often, the peritoneal catheter needs to be removed for a cure.

Candida species are the most common fungal infections and respond poorly to antifungal agents. Therefore, early catheter removal is the recommended therapy for most fungal peritonitis. Peritonitis due to unusual organisms such as mycrobacteria is rare but has been reported in patients from endemic areas.

True 'culture-negative' (aseptic) peritonitis, which also is uncommon with good culture techniques, may be due to chemicals, plasticizer, endotoxin, and the coincidental administration of antibiotics. Eosinophilic peritonitis is an asymptomatic, culture-negative condition of unknown cause that is associated with a cloudy dialysate consisting mainly of eosinophils and usually occurs during the first month after the catheter insertion. Intraperitoneal administration of Vancomycin has been associated with pain and cloudy fluid.

Diagnosis of peritonitis

To make a clinical diagnosis of peritonitis, two of the following three criteria in any combination are required:

(1) Signs and symptoms of peritoneal inflammation such as onset of abdominal pain, rebound tenderness, etc.

(2) Cloudy dialysis solution containing greater than 100 cells/μl, predominantly polymorphonuclear cells. The cell count in an uninfected drained dialysis solution from a CAPD patient is usually less than 50 cells/μl. The majority of these cells are macrophages and monocytes. In IPD patients, the fluid removed at the initiation of dialysis usually has higher cell counts (up to 1000 cells/μl) than CAPD patient fluid.

(3) Identification of organisms either on Gram stain or culture from the drained dialysis solution.

> It is unusual to find bacteremia during CAPD-associated peritonitis and, hence, positive blood culture during an episode should alert for an additional source of infection.

Most peritonitis episodes are mild and can be treated at home. Hypotension is a sign of serious peritonitis and requires aggressive management. Usually, the incubation period for bacterial peritonitis is 24 to 48 hours from the time of contamination. The symptoms and signs resolve quickly after therapy has begun. Slow response or nonresolution of peritonitis after therapy has begun usually indicates either an inappropriate choice of antibiotic or peritonitis due to a source of infection in the

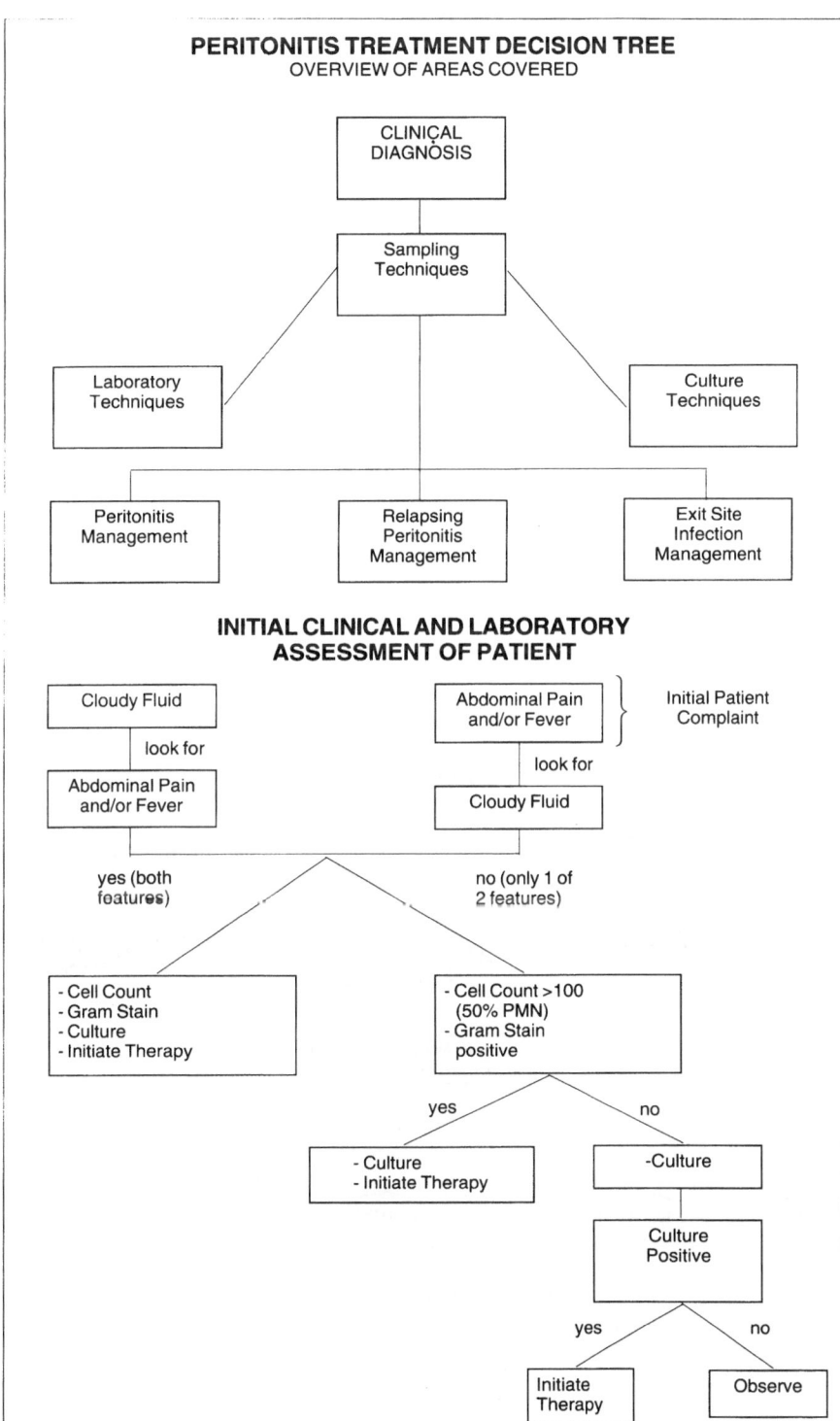

PERITONITIS TREATMENT DECISION TREE
OVERVIEW OF AREAS COVERED

CLINICAL
DIAGNOSIS

Sampling
Techniques

Laboratory
Techniques

Culture
Techniques

Peritonitis
Management

Relapsing
Peritonitis
Management

Exit Site
Infection
Management

**INITIAL CLINICAL AND LABORATORY
ASSESSMENT OF PATIENT**

Cloudy Fluid

Abdominal Pain
and/or Fever

Initial Patient
Complaint

look for

look for

Abdominal Pain
and/or Fever

Cloudy Fluid

yes (both
features)

no (only 1 of
2 features)

- Cell Count
- Gram Stain
- Culture
- Initiate Therapy

- Cell Count >100
  (50% PMN)
- Gram Stain
  positive

yes

no

- Culture
- Initiate Therapy

-Culture

Culture
Positive

yes

no

Initiate
Therapy

Observe

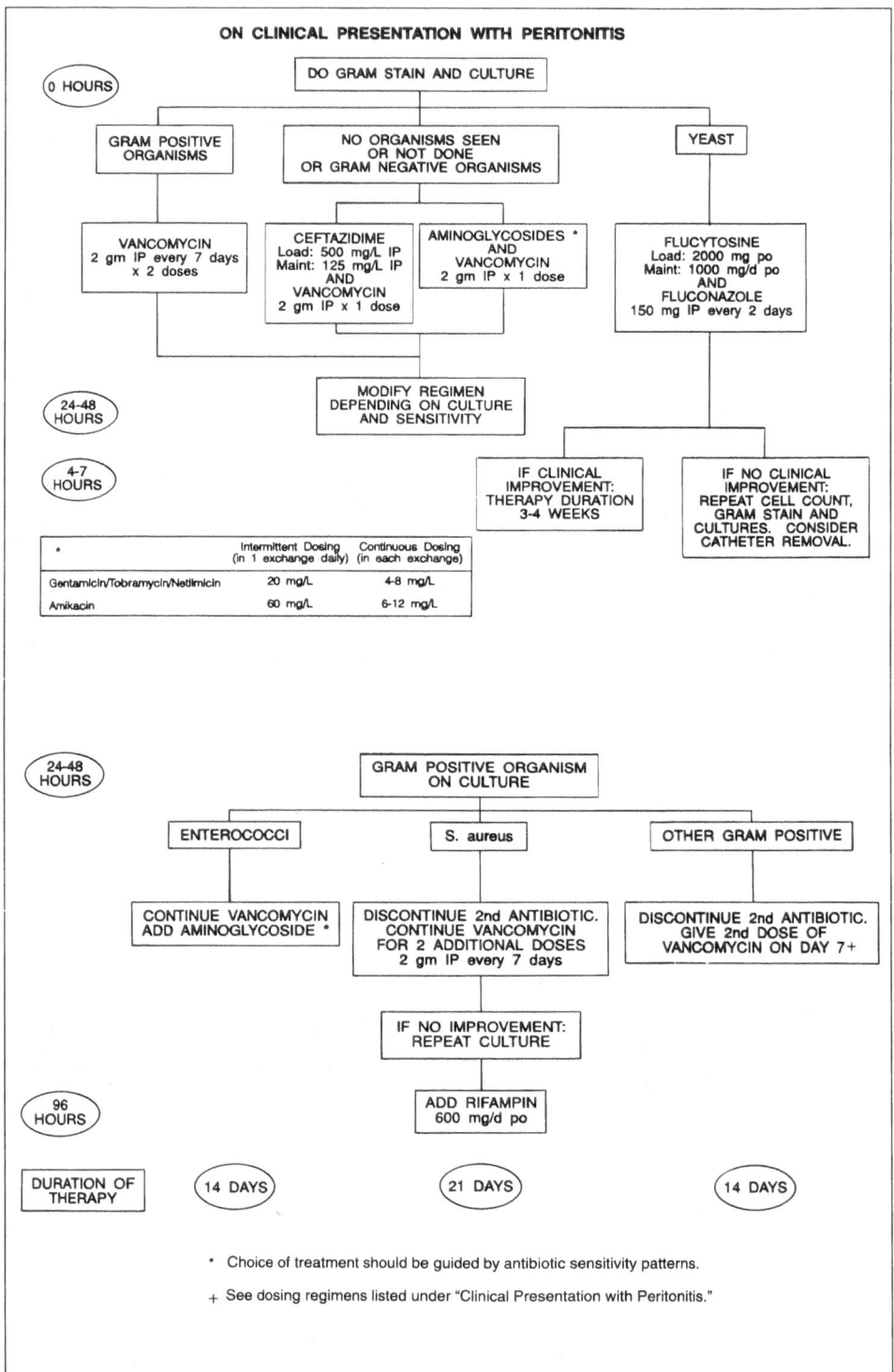

ON CLINICAL PRESENTATION WITH PERITONITIS

0 HOURS → DO GRAM STAIN AND CULTURE

- GRAM POSITIVE ORGANISMS
- NO ORGANISMS SEEN OR NOT DONE OR GRAM NEGATIVE ORGANISMS
- YEAST

GRAM POSITIVE ORGANISMS:
VANCOMYCIN
2 gm IP every 7 days
x 2 doses

NO ORGANISMS SEEN OR NOT DONE OR GRAM NEGATIVE ORGANISMS:
CEFTAZIDIME
Load: 500 mg/L IP
Maint: 125 mg/L IP
AND
VANCOMYCIN
2 gm IP x 1 dose

AMINOGLYCOSIDES *
AND
VANCOMYCIN
2 gm IP x 1 dose

YEAST:
FLUCYTOSINE
Load: 2000 mg po
Maint: 1000 mg/d po
AND
FLUCONAZOLE
150 mg IP every 2 days

24-48 HOURS → MODIFY REGIMEN DEPENDING ON CULTURE AND SENSITIVITY

4-7 HOURS

IF CLINICAL IMPROVEMENT:
THERAPY DURATION
3-4 WEEKS

IF NO CLINICAL IMPROVEMENT:
REPEAT CELL COUNT, GRAM STAIN AND CULTURES. CONSIDER CATHETER REMOVAL.

*	Intermittent Dosing (in 1 exchange daily)	Continuous Dosing (in each exchange)
Gentamicin/Tobramycin/Netilmicin	20 mg/L	4-8 mg/L
Amikacin	60 mg/L	6-12 mg/L

24-48 HOURS → GRAM POSITIVE ORGANISM ON CULTURE

- ENTEROCOCCI
- S. aureus
- OTHER GRAM POSITIVE

ENTEROCOCCI:
CONTINUE VANCOMYCIN
ADD AMINOGLYCOSIDE *

S. aureus:
DISCONTINUE 2nd ANTIBIOTIC.
CONTINUE VANCOMYCIN
FOR 2 ADDITIONAL DOSES
2 gm IP every 7 days

OTHER GRAM POSITIVE:
DISCONTINUE 2nd ANTIBIOTIC.
GIVE 2nd DOSE OF
VANCOMYCIN ON DAY 7+

IF NO IMPROVEMENT:
REPEAT CULTURE

96 HOURS

ADD RIFAMPIN
600 mg/d po

DURATION OF THERAPY   14 DAYS   21 DAYS   14 DAYS

* Choice of treatment should be guided by antibiotic sensitivity patterns.

+ See dosing regimens listed under "Clinical Presentation with Peritonitis."

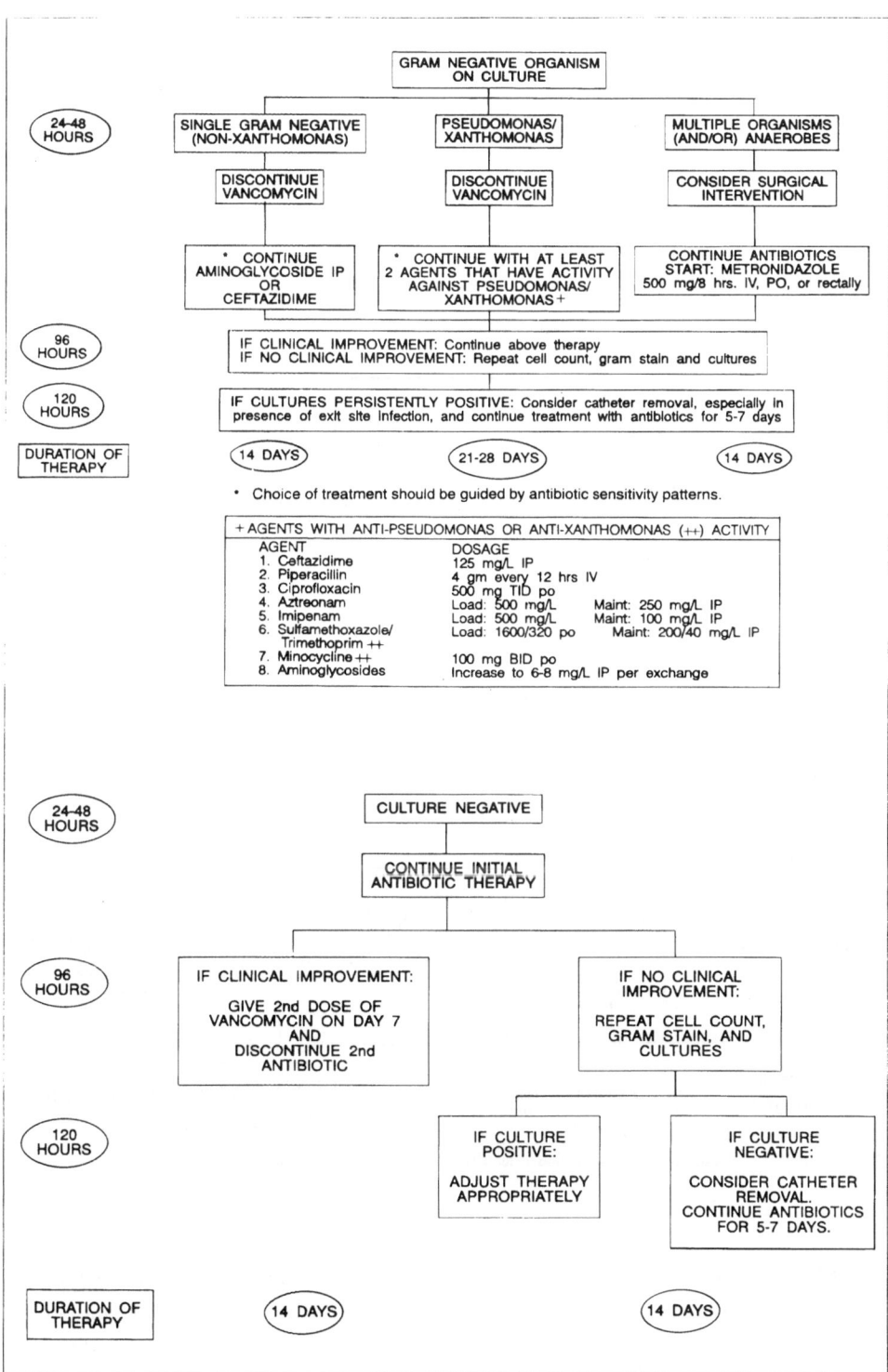

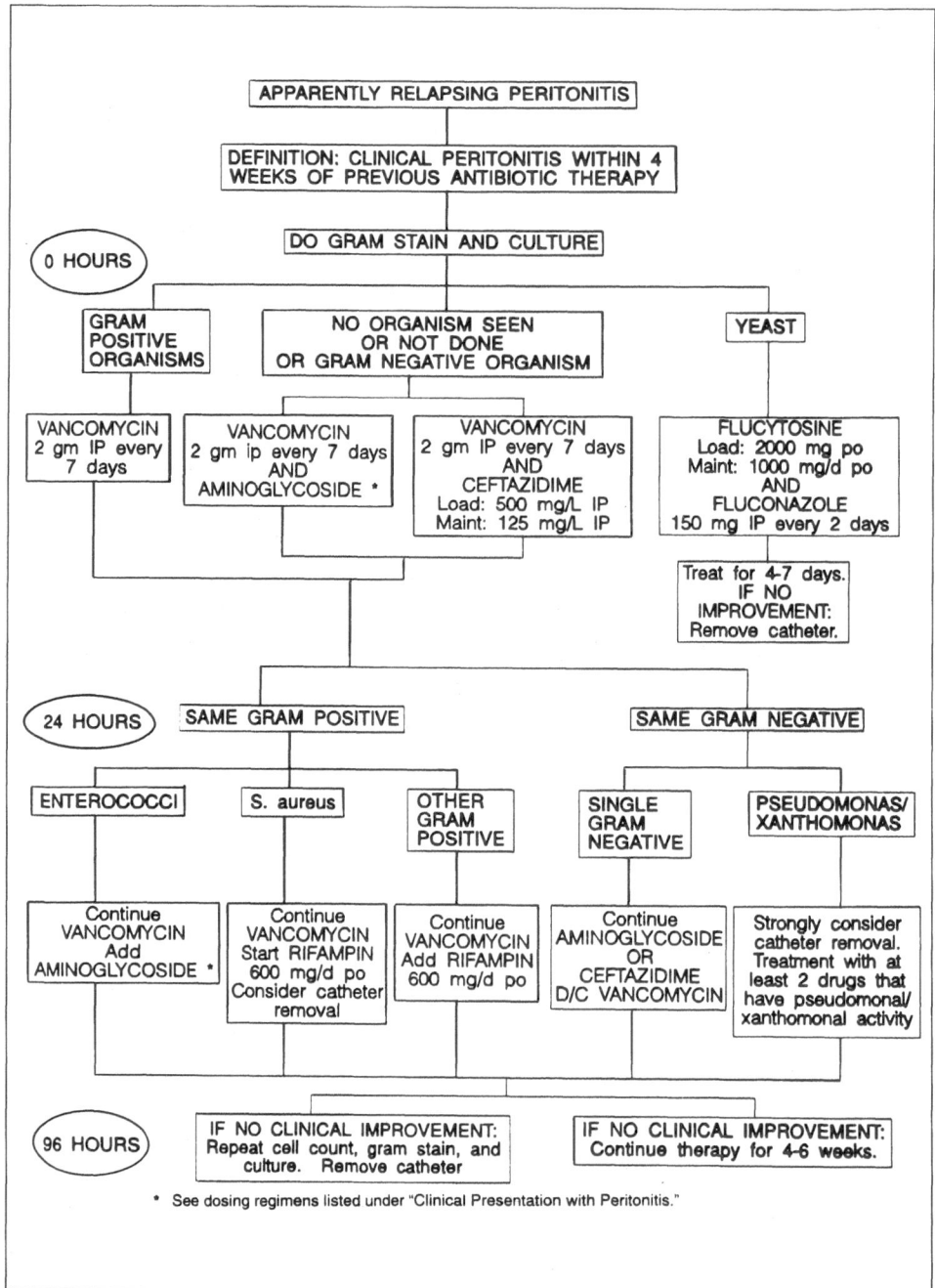

Figure 36: Peritonitis management decision tree as recommended by the Ad Hoc Advisory Committee on Peritonitis Management (1992). (Reproduced with permission from Keane WF, et al. Peritoneal dialysis related peritonitis treatment recommendations. Peritoneal Dialysis International, 1993; 13: 14-28.)

vicinity of the exit or in the tunnel. Peritonitis due to multiple organisms is indicative of a bowel source of the infection.

Management of peritonitis

The Ad Hoc Advisory Committee on Peritonitis Management[1] recommendations for the management of peritonitis are depicted in Figure 36.

In order to establish an accurate diagnosis, a large volume of cloudy dialysis solution should be sent for both Gram stain and culture as early as possible. Gram stain from the sediment of cloudy dialysis solution identifies micro-organisms only in 20 to 30% of cases. Most culture methods currently employ a concentration, filtration, or centrifugation method. Standard culture methods have to be modified by filtration or centrifugation to remove antibiotics from the solution if a patient is being treated with an antibiotic at the time of the collection of dialysis solution.

Early treatment

Once the diagnosis of peritonitis is suspected and the above-mentioned diagnostic work is completed, the following steps of treatment are initiated either at home by the patient or in the hospital by a PD nurse. One to three exchanges (preferably using 1.5% dextrose dialysis solution) in succession are carried out as rapidly as possible, without the addition of antibiotics or insulin in the case of diabetics. These rapid exchanges allow for the wash out of mediators of inflammations from the peritoneal cavity and rapid relief of peritoneal pain. The transfer set may be changed within the first 24 hours of onset, although there is no strong evidence to require such a step.

Fresh dialysis solution is medicated with an aminoglycoside (Tobramycin 1.7 mg/kg body weight), a cephalosporin (cephalothin or cephazolin 1 gm/2 liter solution) and heparin 1000 U/2 liter and infused into the peritoneal cavity and allowed to remain for 6 hours. Alternatively, a gram of intravenous vancomycin infused slowly is an equally effective alternative to cephalosporin. The vancomycin can also be given intraperitoneally but at a higher dose (2 g). The initial choice of antibiotics is made to cover a wide spectrum of organisms.

Each subsequent bag of 2-liter dialysis solution for exchanges contains

[1] Ad Hoc Advisory Committee on Peritonitis Management: See Keane WF, et al. Peritoneal dialysis related peritonitis treatment. Peritoneal Dialysis International 1993; 13:14-28).

TABLE 21. CAPD peritonitis treatment recommendations. Pharmacokinetics of antibiotics in CAPD patients and proposed regimens for the treatment of CAPD peritonitis

| | Half-life (H) | | | Dose (per 70 kg adult)* | | |
| | | | | | Maintenance | |
	Normal	ESRD	CAPD	Initial (mg/2 liter bag)	Intermittent mg/2 liter bag per dosing interval	Continuous (mg/2 liter bag)
Aminoglycosides						
Amikacin	1.6	39	40	500	150/d	12–15
Gentamicin	2.2	53	32	70–140	50/d	8–16
Netilmicin	2.1	42	18	70–140	60/d	8–16
Tobramycin	2.5	58	36	70–140	50/d	8–16
Cephalosporins						
First generation						
Cefazolin	2.2	28	30	500–1000	1000/d	250–500
Cefonicid	4.0	68	50	250	ND	50
Cephalothin	0.2	3.7	ND	1000	ND	200
Cephradine	0.9	12	ND	500	ND	250
Cephalexin	0.8	19	9	1000 PO	500/QID PO	NA
Second generation						
Cefamandole	1.0	10	8.0	1000	1000/d	500
Cefmenoxime	1.3	11.3	6.0	2000	1000/d	100
Cefotiam	1.0	7.0	8.0	1000	1000/d	50
Cefoxitin	0.8	20	15	1000	ND	200
Cefuroxime	1.3	18	15	1000	ND	150–400
Third generation						
Cefixime	3.2	11.5	15	400 PO	400/d PO	NA
Cefoperazone	1.8	2.3	2.2	2000	ND	400–1000
Cefotaxime	0.9	2.5	2.4	2000	2000/d	500
Cefsulodin	1.8	11	11	1000	1000/d	50
Ceftazidime	1.8	26	13	1000	500/d	100–250
Ceftizoxime	1.6	28	11	1000	1000/d	250
Ceftriaxone	8.0	15	12	1000	1000/d	250–500
Moxalactam	2.2	20	16	1000	1000/d	350
Penicillins						
Azlocillin	0.9	5.1	ND	500	ND	500
Mezlocillin	1.0	4.3	ND	3000 IV	3000/BIC IV	500

Piperacillin	1.2	3.9	ND	4000 IV	4000/BID IV	500
Ticarcillin	1.2	15	ND	1000–2000	2000/BID	250
Quinolones						
Ciprofloxacin	4.0	8.0	10	750 PO	750/BID PO	50
Fleroxacin	13	27	27	800 PO	400/d PO	NA
Ofloxacin	7.0	30	25	400 PO	200/d PO	NA
Vancomycin and others						
Vancomycin	6.9	161	92	1000–2000	1–2000/7 d	30–50
Teicoplanin	50	260	260	400	400/BID	40[a]
Aztreonam	2.0	7.0	7.1	1000	ND	500
Clindamycin	2.8	2.8	300	ND	300	
Erythromycin	2.1	4.0	ND	ND	500/QID PO	150
Metronidazole	7.9	7.7	11	500/TID PO/IV	ND	
Rifaampin	4.0	8.0	ND	600 PO	600/d PO	NA
Antifungal agents						
Amphotericin	360	360	ND	NA	20–30/d IV	2–8
Flucytosine	4.2	115	ND	2000–3000 PO	1000/d PO	NA
				200	400/d	100–200
Ketoconazole	2.0	1.8	2.4	400 PO	200–800/d PO	NA
Miconazole	24	25	ND	200	ND	100–200
Combinations						
Ampicillin	1.3	15	9.5	1000–2000	100/BID	100
Sulbactam	1.0	19	9.7	1000–2000	1000/BID	100
Imipenem	0.9	3.0	3.3	500–1000	500/BID	100–200
Cilistatin	0.8	15	9	500–1000	500/BID	100–200
Sulfamethoxazole	10	13	14	1600 PO	1600/1–2 d PO	200–400
Trimethoprim	14	33	34	320 PO	320/1–2 d PO	40–80

* The route of administration is intraperitoneal unless otherwise specified. The pharmacokinetic data and proposed dosage regimens presented here are based on published literature reviewed through January 1989.
There is no evidence that mixing different antibiotics in dialysis fluid (except for aminoglycosides and penicillins) is deleterious for the drugs or patients. Do not use the same syringe to mix antibiotics.

a This is in each bag × 7 days, then in 2 bags/day × 7 days and then in 1 bag/day × 7 days.

ESRD = Creatinine clearance < 10 ml/min, patient not on dialysis: NA = Not applicable: ND = No data; IV = Intravenous; PO = Oral; d = Once a day; BID = Twice a day; TID = Three times a day; QID = Four times a day.

(Reproduced with permission Keane WF, et al. Peritoneal dialysis related peritonitis treatment recommendations. Peritoneal Dialysis International, 1993,13:14-28.)

16 mg of tobramycin, 200–500 mg of a cephalosporin, and 1000 U of heparin. Tobramycin and cephalosporin should not be mixed in the same syringe but can be mixed safely in the same dialysate bag. This regime is continued until the results of Gram stain and/or culture and antibiotic sensitivity are available. Appropriate changes in the antibiotics are then made if necessary. In the case of a Gram-positive organism peritonitis, it is not necessary to continue with the administration of the aminoglycoside. The half-lives, loading and maintenance doses of different antibiotics are listed in the Table 21.

The resolution of peritonitis is monitored clinically and with periodic dialysate white cell counts. If the peritonitis is resolving, antibiotics are discontinued 7 to 10 days after the start of therapy. The peritonitis treatment protocol is modified for fungal, tuberculous, 'surgical' or multiple-organism peritonitis, or peritonitis following tunnel abscess or severe exit-site infection. In most of these special situations, treatment includes removal of the peritoneal catheter, systemic administration of the appropriate antibacterial or antifungal agents, and drainage of the abscess, if present.

Peritonitis during APD is treated with loading doses of intravenous antibiotics. Additionally, during the dialysis exchanges, maintenance antibiotics and heparin in the dosage recommended for CAPD patients are added to the dialysis solution. Resolution of peritonitis is monitored with predialysis cell counts. IPD patients receive antibiotics intraperitoneally during the dialysis, and they may not need any antibiotics in between the dialysis days. Patients on CCPD receive intraperitoneal antibiotics in every exchange including the long-dwell daytime exchanges.

Recurrent peritonitis, not responding to appropriate antibiotics, is treated with catheter removal. In such cases, a new catheter is usually inserted after 10 to 15 days, by which time peritonitis is usually resolved. Successful catheter reinsertion may be carried out at the time of the catheter removal, but at the risk of reinfection of the new catheter. Patients in whom the catheter is removed without a replacement, are maintained on hemodialysis using a subclavian or femoral access.

Absorption of antibiotics from the dialysis solution to serum is rapid. Therefore, in most cases it is not necessary to give the antibiotics intravenously. The outcome of peritonitis treatment with intraperitoneal or intravenous antibiotics is comparable and therefore the choice of one method versus another should be tailored to the patient and facility situations.

During peritonitis, probably because of an increased blood flow through the peritoneum, peritoneal clearances of large and small molecules increase and also glucose absorption increases. As a result, patients may develop hypophosphatemia, hypokalemia, and hypoproteinemia and also

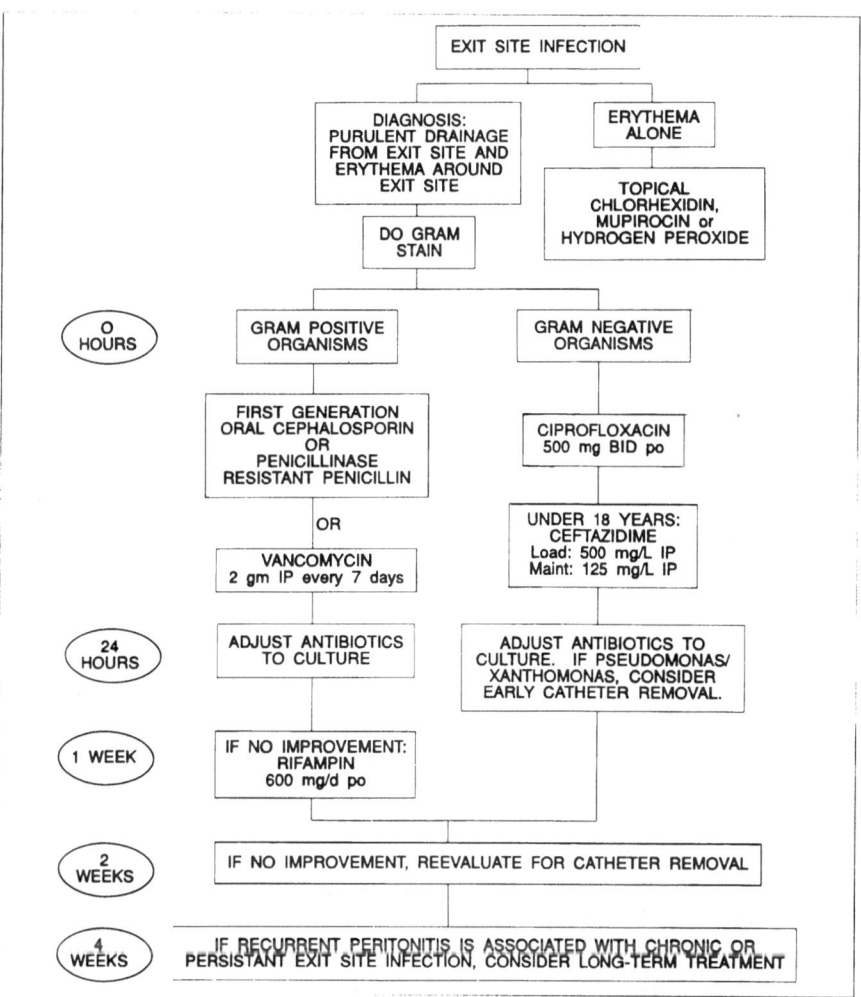

Figure 37: Exit-site infection management as recommended by the Ad Hoc Advisory Committee on Peritonitis Management 1992. (Reproduced with permission from Keane WF, et al. Peritoneal dialysis related peritonitis treatment recommendations. Peritoneal Dialysis International; 1993; 13:14-28.)

impaired ultrafiltration. If peritonitis leads to extensive adhesions, as can occur after fecal, pseudomonas, or *S. aureus* peritonitis, the peritoneum may permanently lose its capacity to ultrafilter and transfer solutes and peritoneal dialysis may have to be abandoned.

For patients severely ill with peritonitis, hospitalization is indicated. A course of oral or parenteral rifampin is indicated for patients with persistent or recurrent *S. aureus* infection. In these patients, defective intracellular bactericidal properties of peritoneal macrophages allow persistence of viable organisms inside the cell. Rifampin penetrates these cells and eradicates the bacteria. Accidental contaminations are treated with a change of transfer set followed by either a course of cephalosporin or a single intravenous injection of a gram of vancomycin. After the treatment of peritonitis and before the patient goes home, a CAPD nurse should review the patient's technique in an attempt to identify and to correct errors in technique which might have contributed to the peritonitis.

> Antibiotic prophylaxis for peritonitis is not recommended because it favors the emergence of resistant organisms.

Encapsulating or sclerosing peritonitis (i.e., the formation of a dense layer of fibroconnective tissue on the peritoneal membrane, encapsulating the bowel like a cocoon) may appear several months or years after cessation of either IPD or CAPD. The disease progresses slowly and may remain asymptomatic for a long time; however, rapid progression also has been described. Presenting symptoms may include loss of ultrafiltration capacity (with rapid glucose absorption initially and with slow glucose absorption later), recurrent abdominal pain, intermittent vomiting, and eventually, partial or complete small bowel obstruction. Peritoneal clearances of solutes usually remain at an acceptable level but may decrease in later stages. Such sclerosis is a serious complication with a high incidence of fatal outcomes. Most deaths result from severe malnutrition, sepsis, and bowel-related surgical complications. Fortunately, the incidence of this problem in CAPD patients is extremely low.

The cause of peritoneal membrane sclerosis is unknown. Afflicted patients have a higher frequency of certain 'risk' factors – namely, recurrent severe peritonitis treated with numerous antibiotics, use of acetate-containing solution, high use of hypertonic solutions because of loss of ultrafiltration capacity, use of chlorhexidine antiseptic solutions, and use of beta-blockers. It is noteworthy that this complication is extremely rare in those who have used only lactate-containing dialysis solutions manufactured in North America. Because we lack a proper understanding of this disease process, no definitive strategy has evolved to prevent it.

The management of exit-site infection is depicted in Figure 37. A traumatized exit site is prone to develop infection. A prohylactic antibiotic in such a situation may prevent serious infection.

9 COMPLICATIONS DURING PERITONEAL DIALYSIS

The complications seen during peritoneal dialysis are either modified uremic organ dysfunctions (Figure 38) or have arisen as a result of peritoneal dialysis (Figure 39).

Uremic organ dysfunction during CAPD

Nutritional problems

Following the initiation of CAPD in ESRD patients, an anabolic state is achieved due to the continuous supply of energy in the form of glucose.

This anabolic state is evidenced by weight gain, improvement of anemia, and normalization of acid-base and electrolyte status. But, the continuous supply of 100–200 g/day of glucose through the dialysis solution may predispose to hypertriglyceridemia, hyperinsulinemia, carbohydrate intolerance, and obesity in some patients.

The continuous supply of glucose is offset by the continuous loss of protein in the drained dialysis solution, especially during an episode of peritonitis.

In a stable CAPD patient, the protein and amino acid losses per day averages 6–12 g. In order to compensate for such losses, these patients may need to consume a dietary protein of at least 1 g/kg body weight/day. Most CAPD patients maintain serum protein and albumin levels that are

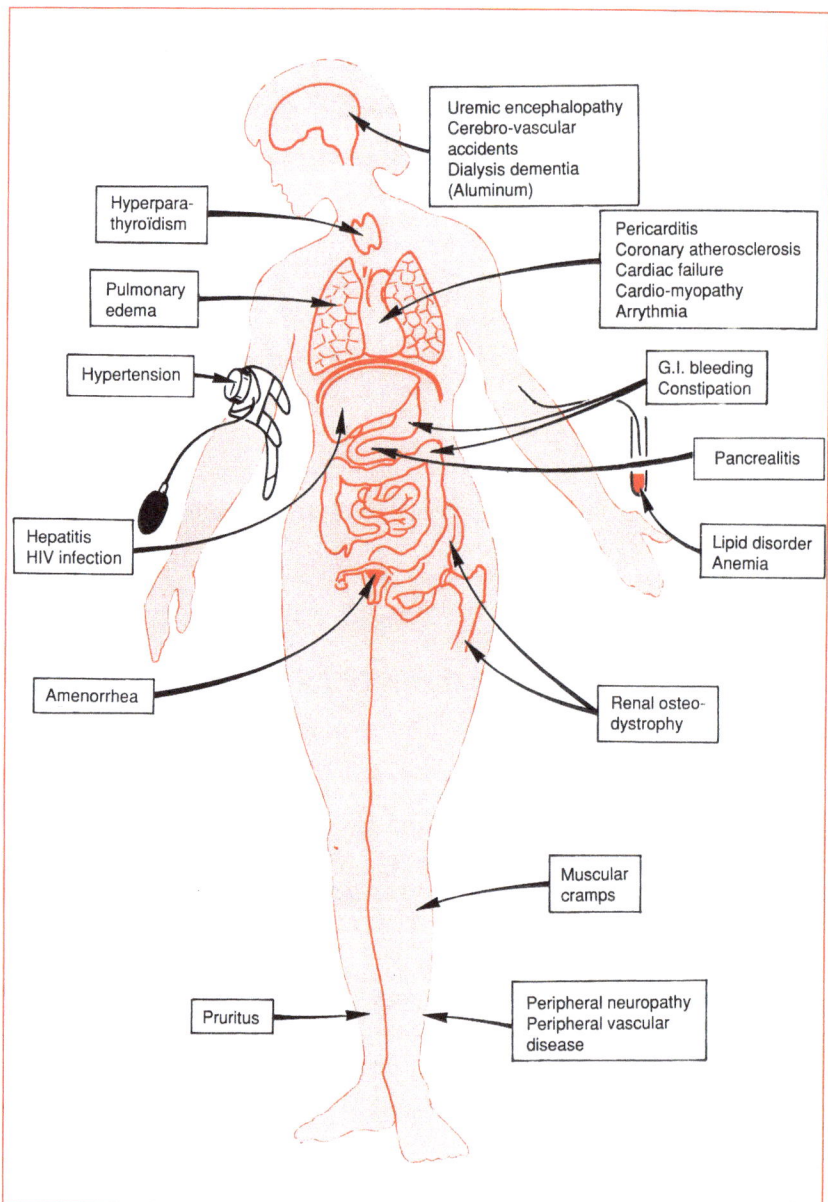

Figure 38: Uremic organ dysfunctions during CAPD.

slightly lower than the normal range. Abnormal plasma amino acid levels (high concentrations of several nonessential amino acids and low concentrations of essential amino acids) and muscle-free amino acids (low taurine levels) seen in the nondialyzed uremics seem to persist despite ade-

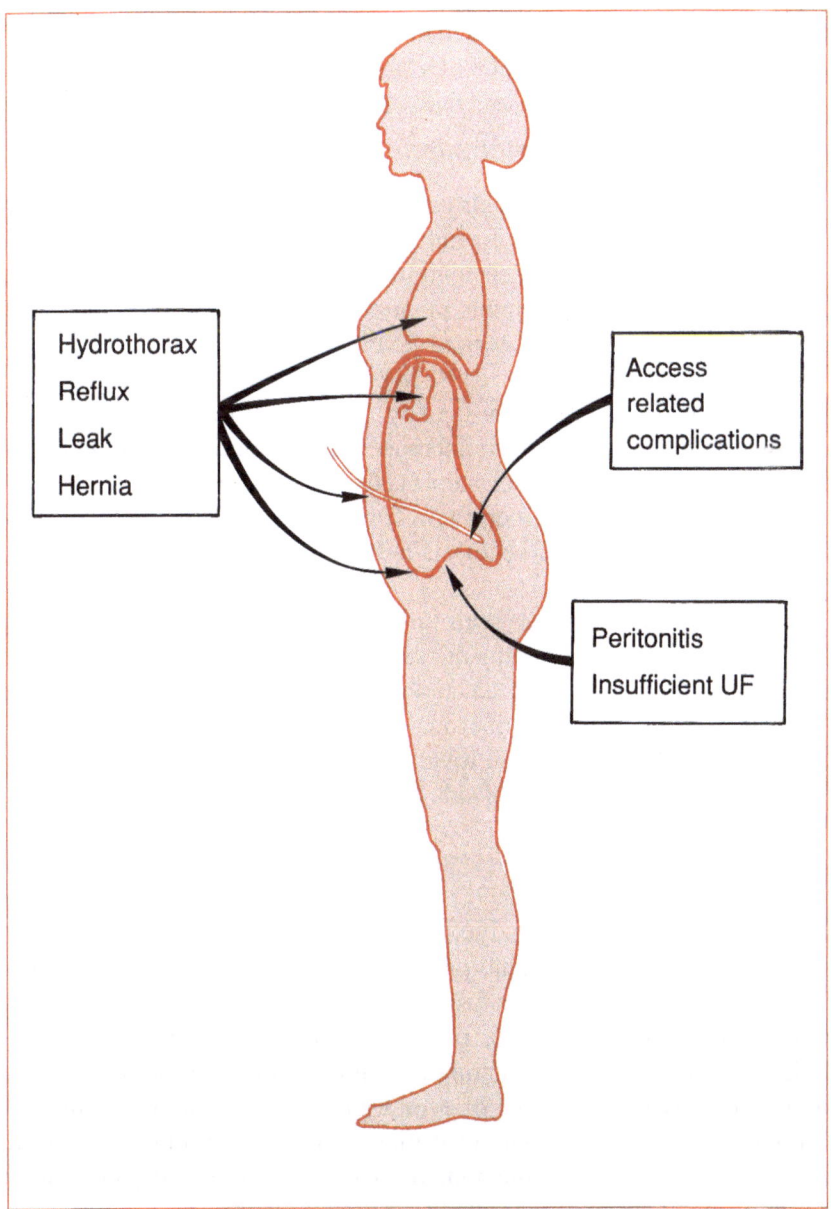

Figure 39: Technique related complications of PD.

quate dialysis. Water-soluble vitamins, B complex and folic acid, are also lost during CAPD, and the blood levels of these compounds are often low without supplementation.

Overall, CAPD patients are in a state of net anabolism during the first few years of therapy. Some degree of malnutrition is seen in about 8–30% of CAPD patients who have been on therapy for longer than three months.

Abnormalities of lipid metabolism

Although serum cholesterol levels are higher in CAPD patients compared to hemodialysis patients, the levels are marginally higher than normal levels. Serum triglyceride levels tend to be more variable but, in general, most CAPD patients have levels persistently above the normal range; some have 5 to 10 times the normal levels. Exposure to drugs, e.g., androgen, beta-blockers, known to cause hypertriglyceridemia, may aggravate the problem. Elevated very low-density lipoprotein (VLDL) cholesterol and triglyceride during uremia increase further during CAPD. High-density lipoprotein (HDL)-cholesterol is low initially and remains low through the therapy. Loss of lipoprotein fractions into the dialysis solution occurs, but minimally. The synthesis is higher than the loss, causing increased levels.

Treatment of lipid disorders seen in patients during CAPD is difficult, but nonpharmacological treatment, such as dietary counseling, weight loss, exercise, and restriction of alcohol intake can be beneficial. Drug therapy is associated with numerous toxic side effects. However, low-dose treatment with some lipid lowering drugs may be tried with close monitoring for the occurrence of side effects.

Hematological problems

Anemia during peritoneal dialysis is less severe than during hemodialysis, probably because patients on peritoneal dialysis do not lose blood as do those on hemodialysis. Transfusion requirements of patients on peritoneal dialysis are lower than for those on chronic hemodialysis. During CAPD, the improvement in anemia is striking, and in some patients the hemoglobin may reach normal or even higher levels. The mechanism of this improvement is unknown but it may represent the removal of toxic substances, which suppress the bone marrow's response to erythropoietin and reduce the life span of red cells.

Preliminary experience with subcutaneous erythropoietin in CAPD patients indicates a lower dose requirement to achieve a similar response compared to hemodialysis patients.

The hemoglobin-oxygen dissociation curve has been demonstrated to be shifted to the right in CAPD patients, indicating a better oxygenation of the tissues. Platelet dysfunction and prolonged bleeding time associated with uremia are reversed with CAPD, probably due to removal of uremic toxins.

Hypertension

Hypertension is common in patients starting dialysis, and usually it can be controlled by reducing total body sodium and by ultrafiltration.

> Most patients, even those suffering from malignant hypertension, become normotensive within one to two months of starting CAPD and many may become hypotensive (interestingly, the blood pressure returns to normal at a time when dry body weight is increasing).

If the patient becomes hypotensive, administration of sodium chloride by mouth while simultaneously keeping the body weight normal by dialysis usually returns the blood pressure to normal. The pressure response to infusion of angiotensin is diminished in hypotensive CAPD patients, probably as a result of total body sodium depletion. Correction of anemia with erythropoietin increases blood pressure, especially after a rapid correction.

Renal osteodystrophy

CAPD removes some parathyroid hormone fractions (iPTH), but does not substantially reduce the plasma levels of parathyroid hormone. iPTH decreases only when its secretion is suppressed by an increase in serum calcium or high serum levels of calcitriol. At the initiation of CAPD, most patients have histological evidence of bone disease, either of high turnover (osteitis fibrosa cystica with increased osteoclasts and osteoblasts, peritubular fibrosis, tunnelling resorption, and formation of woven bone) or low turnover (mineralization defect, thin osteoid seams, decreased numbers of osteoclasts and osteoblasts and absent aluminum staining). To decrease the serum iPTH and stimulate healing of the osteitis fibrosa, the serum calcium must be maintained at slightly hypercalcemic levels (10.5–11 mg/dl. The incidence of hypercalcemia (levels above 12 mg %) in CAPD patients using calcium (carbonate or acetate) as a phosphate binding agent is approximately 30%. Use of lower calcium dialysis solutions (2.5 mEg/liter) can prevent such hypercalcemia. Aplastic bone disease is a low-turnover condition frequently found in CAPD patients, even in the absence of aluminum toxicity. It is characterized by a low PTH level and a tendency for hypercalcemia.

By itself, CAPD does not normalize the serum phosphate levels but requires use of phosphate binders. Aluminum binders may cause toxicity. To avoid such problems, calcium carbonate (3–6 gm/day) is used as a phosphate binder. It is important that patients take calcium with meals, otherwise calcium binding may be minimal and hypercalcemia may occur more. Incidence of hypercalcemia is reduced by the use of low calcium (2.5 mEq/liter) dialysis solution. When serum phosphorus is 6 mg/dl or more, one must avoid using vitamin D or its metabolites to prevent a further increase in the serum calcium and phosphorus and, thus, soft-tissue calcification.

It has now become clear that long-term use of aluminum-containing phosphate binders may cause significant aluminum accumulation in the body, leading to aluminum toxicity (aluminum-induces osteomalacia or dialysis dementia), hence, their use should be severely curtailed. Calcium carbonate is an effective phosphate binder in most patients.

Neurological complications

Nerve conduction velocities do not decrease in patients undergoing either hemodialysis or peritoneal dialysis, except in those who are underdialyzed or severely malnourished. Studies in patients on CAPD for periods of up to 2 years show no deterioration in nerve conduction velocities.

The causes of confusional states in peritoneal dialysis patients include underdialysis, hypercalcemia or hypoglycemias, altered electrolyte abnormalities, drug toxicity, and aluminum intoxication with encephalopathy. Dialysis dementia occurs very infrequently in peritoneal dialysis patients. An association has been observed between dialysis dementia and serum aluminum level. Unexplained increases in serum aluminum may be observed in some patients, which may relate to use of calcium citrate; citrate enhances aluminum absorption from the gut. Similarly, dialysis disequilibrium is rarely seen with peritoneal dialysis patients because urea removal during PD is slow.

Pericarditis

The frequency of pericarditis in ESRD patients undergoing any form of dialysis has ranged from 15 to 20%. However, the incidence is low in CAPD patients (< 5%). Clinically, pericarditis presents with chest pain, a pericardial friction rub, low-grade temperature, and mild leukocytosis. Tamponade can be controlled by needle pericardiocentesis, but, if it is recurrent, one proceeds to surgical pericardiectomy. Pericarditis without tamponade generally responds to conservative management, namely increased dialysis, salt restriction, and strict control of fluid intake. The incidence of pericarditis with CAPD is extremely low and, when it occurs, it is usually due to underdialysis by a noncompliant patient.

Vascular problems

CAPD may have a deleterious effect in the presence of generalized atherosclerosis with compromised circulation to the lower extremities and partial occlusions in iliofemoral vessels: reduced perfusion as a result of hypotension, which is not uncommon during CAPD, can provoke ischemic complications. Such patients may require corrective or palliative surgery to relieve their symptoms.

CAPD patients are noted to have a large number of cardiovascular and cerebrovascular problems, such as recurrent angina, arrhythmias, acute myocardial infarction, transient ischemic attacks, and complete strokes, but no one has yet defined the contribution of CAPD to their pathogenesis. Some have suggested that the increased incidence of cardiovascular and cerebrovascular complications in dialysis patients is due to accelerated atherosclerosis associated with hypertriglyceridemia and low levels of high-density liproprotein fractions. However, many patients coming to CAPD are older and, hence, have heart and brain complications; even so, it is possible that CAPD may accelerate these complications.

Endocrine function

Decrease in total T_4 and total T_3, probably related to changes in thyroid-binding globulin or an altered affinity between thyroxine and its binding globulin, are frequently observed. An increased amount of circulating reverse T_3 is also frequently noted. The TSH is at the high normal or elevated range with a blunted response to TRH stimulation.

Serum levels of prolactin are elevated in CAPD patients and hyperprolactinemia has been identified as one of the many causes of infertility and sexual dysfunction that occurs in uremia. Basal levels of growth hormone are not significantly different between CAPD and hemodialysis patients. The growth-hormone response to insulin induced hypoglycemia is greater in HD patients than those on CAPD. The levels of follicle-stimulating hormone and luteinizing hormone are elevated in both dialysis groups to an equal degree. Testosterone levels are lower than normal in male CAPD patients. Many women on CAPD have normal menstruation with ovulatory cycles, and some have even become pregnant.

Acquired cystic disease of the kidney

The prevalence of acquired renal cystic disease seems to be similar in both hemodialysis and CAPD patients. The cystic lesions can occasionally have malignant transformation and cause retroperitoneal bleeding.

Complications due to peritoneal dialysis

The technique complications are related to (1) access, (2) solution, and (3) increased intra-abdominal pressure. Access related complications have been discussed under the access section. Peritonitis can cause acute ultrafiltration failure. Peritonitis and related complications have been discussed in the chapter dealing with peritonitis and ultrafiltration failure is discussed in this chapter.

Pressure-related complications

The continuous presence of a large volume of dialysis solution in the peritoneal cavity increases the intra-abdominal pressure which further increases with such activities as walking and jogging. Coughing and straining generates the highest intra-abdominal pressure.

> Continuous elevation of intra-abdominal pressure predisposes to abdominal hernias (incisional, inguinal, diaphragmatic, or umbilical) and dialysate leaks, especially in older patients with or without previous surgical scars.

Edema of the labia majoris, scrotum, and penis are distressing complications which occur due to dialysis solution leaking through the soft tissue plane from an incision site or from a soft tissue defect in a hernia. The site of leak may be detected by a contrast CAT scan or abdominal isotopic scintigraphy. Minor leaks may stop after transient interruption of CAPD. However, both hernias and persistent leak warrant surgical repair before PD is reinitiated. Peritoneal dialysis may be continued in the supine position if, for any reason, surgery is not feasible. The site of leak may seal if CAPD is temporarily discontinued. During this period, the patient is maintained on supine peritoneal dialysis or hemodialysis. Multiparous females may develop a rectocoele or a cystocoele, with or without uterine prolapse. Symptoms of gastro-esophageal reflux, hiatus hernia, and hemorrhoids are aggravated. Carrying the 2-liter of dialysis solution during upright ambulation exaggerates normal lordotic posture which, in some patients, may cause back pain and aggravate symptoms in people with vertebral disease. In such a situation, nightly peritoneal dialysis should be recommended.

Transdiaphragmatic dialysis solution leak into the pleural cavity is a rare but serious pressure-related complication. High glucose (higher than serum level) and low protein concentrations in the drained pleural fluid are diagnostic. Patients may continue on supine peritoneal dialysis if the communication is small. If the leak is big and causes massive effusion, peritoneal dialysis has to be discontinued. Repair of the defect in the diaphragm, if localized, allows patients to return to peritoneal dialysis. Success of pleurodesis with talc or tetracycline is equivocal and therefore is only attempted in those who are unwilling to transfer to hemodialysis.

Insufficient ultrafiltration

A sudden loss of ultrafiltration is usually first noticed by the patient; the drain bag will have insufficient return of fluid. However, minor change in ultrafiltration volume occurring gradually goes unnoticed by the patient and manifests in fluid retention and edema formation. Different causes of ultrafiltration failure are listed in Table 22.

When a patient complains of insufficient fluid return or edema formation, the catheter function and the residual urine output should be checked before proceeding with the ultrafiltration failure work-up, as detailed in Figure 40.

A transient catheter flow problem due to fibrin clot in the dialysate or external pressure on the catheter from the neighboring structures may slow down the solution return. When such a problem arises, a patient accustomed to draining the solution over a fixed period proceeds to the next

TABLE 22. Causes of insufficient ultrafiltration/fluid retention in patients during CAPD

1. Poorly functioning catheter
   (a) excessive fibrin in the fluid
   (b) external catheter compression
   (c) omental entrapment
2. Dialysis solution leak into the soft-tissue planes
3. Peritoneal membrane function alteration
   (a) transient during bacterial peritonitis
   (b) chemical peritonitis
   (c) sclerosing peritonitis
4. Severe adhesion formation
5. Excessive lymphatic flow

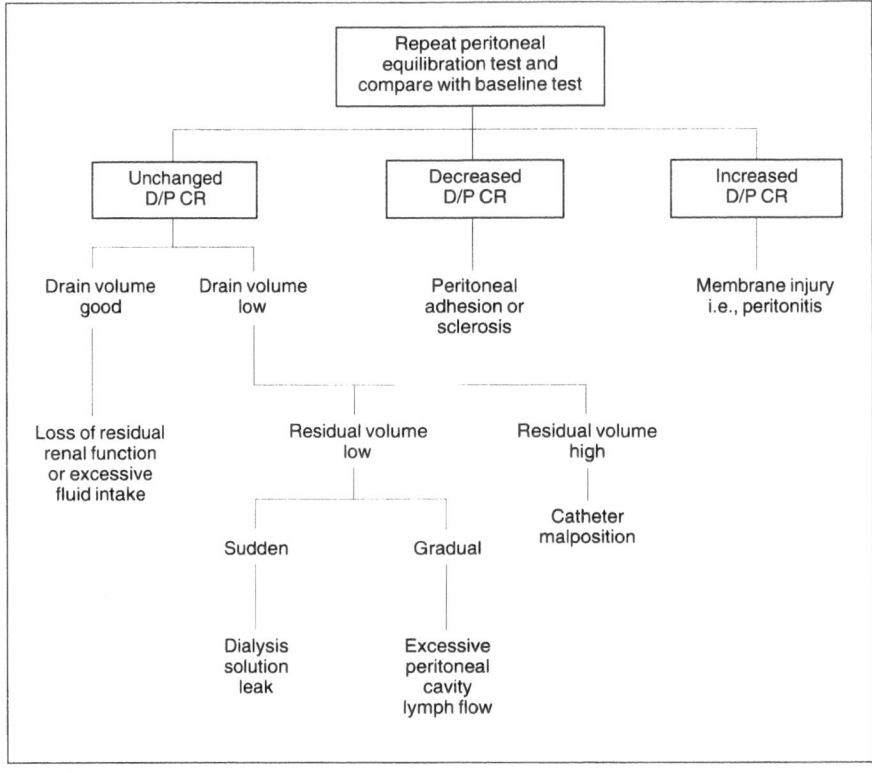

Figure 40: Algorithm for insufficient ultrafiltration in CAPD patients.

exchange without completely draining the peritoneal cavity, resulting in the accumulation of a large residual volume. Restoring the catheter function is all that is required to cure such a problem. The steps of diagnosis of other causes of insufficient ultrafiltration and their management are summarized in Figure 40.

10 PERITONEAL DIALYSIS IN DIABETICS

The many advantages coupled with the encouraging trend for better survival with CAPD and CCPD have made these treatment alternatives very attractive for diabetics requiring dialysis.

Why choose CAPD over other dialysis therapies?

Diabetic patients approaching end stage renal disease suffer from damage to other organs such as eye, heart, bladder, bowel, and nerves.

> In such patients, rapid hemodynamic alterations, as might occur with any intermittent form of dialysis, may cause frequent episodes of hypotension, thus risking coronary or cerebrovascular events.

Acute or prolonged hypotension, as might occur with any intermittent dialysis, may worsen peripheral vascular disease. Peritoneal access is easy to establish and this avoids having to access an atherosclerosed blood vessel. The medical benefits of CAPD for diabetics are listed in Table 23. Besides these medical benefits, there are several socio-economic advantages with CAPD, such as easy adaptation to home dialysis and free mobility. Since

TABLE 23. The medical benefits of CAPD for diabetic ESRD patients

1. Capability to administer intraperitoneal insulin
2. Good blood pressure control
3. Good fluid and electrolyte balance
4. Peritoneal access is easy and does not have to use vascular access

the procedure can be carried out without a machine, CAPD is convenient for free mobility and easy to adapt for home treatment.

For those complicated diabetics who are unsuitable for renal transplantation, CAPD/CCPD is considered appropriate, because it is a slow continuous process and has the potential advantage of reduced cardiovascular stress and stable hemodynamic status. A steady biochemical state, easy control of hypertension and extracellular fluid volume, and the possibility of intraperitoneal insulin administration for blood sugar control are the additional reasons to choose this therapy.

What is the ideal time to initiate dialysis in diabetics?

Because of the frequent association of severe vascular disease and eye complications in diabetic ESRD patients, many prefer to initiate dialysis for them early, at a creatinine clearance of 10 ml/min, a GFR level slightly higher than recommended (5-8 ml/min) for nondiabetic ESRD patients, in the hope of preserving some useful function in these organs. Moreover, a diabetic patient becomes symptomatic with progressive renal failure – probably due to a higher propensity to retain fluid – at a GFR slightly higher than nondiabetics.

Peritoneal access

It is possible to use the catheter for supine peritoneal dialysis immediately after its insertion. This avoids the need for temporary access or preplanned access surgery so often necessary in hemodialysis.

The techniques of catheter insertion, break-in procedure, and post-operative catheter care in diabetics are similar to nondiabetic patients. Infectious and noninfectious catheter complications and catheter survival rates are not different for diabetics compared to nondiabetic patients on peritoneal dialysis. However, the route of insulin delivery seems to influence the incidence of exit-site and/or tunnel infection. Diabetics not using insulin tend to have the lowest rates of exit-site/tunnel infection per patient year (0.4), while patients using subcutaneous insulin experience the highest rate (0.65). Blind patients experience similar rates of exit-site/tunnel infection irrespective of the route of insulin administration. Catheter replacement rates per patient year are similar for all patient groups (0.16 to 0.20).

Is glucose an ideal osmotic agent for diabetic CAPD patients?

Glucose has proved to be an effective osmotic agent for generating ultra-filtration during peritoneal dialysis. An average CAPD patient typically absorbs 100–150 grams of glucose per day during the course of CAPD therapy. However, use of glucose has been associated with numerous undesirable metabolic effects, such as hyperinsulinemia, obesity, hypertriglyceridemia, and premature atherosclerosis. These problems have led to the search for alternative osmotic agents, such as xylitol, amino acids, gelatin, polyglucose, and glycerol. None of the agents tried have the favorable profile of glucose, either because of unacceptable toxicity or prohibitive costs.

Thus, for now, despite several drawbacks, glucose still remains the preferred osmotic agent for peritoneal dialysis.

Dialysis regimens and blood-sugar control

Intermittent peritoneal dialysis (IPD)

Blood-sugar control, while on IPD, is achieved with insulin administered both subcutaneously and intraperitoneally. The amount of insulin administered is adjusted to the individual requirements. On dialysis days, patients are given the usual daily dose of insulin by subcutaneous injection and an additional amount of regular insulin is added to the dialysis solution until the last few exchanges of dialysis. Insulin is omitted from the last few exchanges to prevent post-dialysis hypoglycemia. Insulin requirements, once established, do not usually change unless a complication is encountered.

Retinopathy and neuropathy stabilize in patients on IPD during the course of treatment. Hemoglobin and hematocrit are maintained at satisfactory levels without blood transfusions. Compared to nondiabetics on IPD, diabetic patients experience a higher incidence of peritonitis and hypertension is more common compared to CAPD patients. The majority of the patients die from cardiac and cerebrovascular complications. A significant percentage of patients die suddenly at home, presumably due to a coronary event or from an electrolyte abnormality. The probability of patient survival at 1 and 2 years is 44 and 20%, respectively. Use of IPD has declined since the advent of CAPD in the mid-seventies. However, a variant of IPD with a longer total weekly duration of treatment, i.e. daily nighttime IPD (NIPD), is now used in selected patients who are unsuitable for CAPD. Insulin can be given subcutaneously during daytime hours and in the solutions at night.

Continuous cyclic peritoneal dialysis (CCPD)

Excellent glycemic control can be achieved in the majority of CCPD patients if a regular and predictable caloric intake is maintained. The insulin dose is divided among all the dialysis solution bags depending upon the caloric load. The average intraperitoneal insulin dose required for good control of glycemia has been about three times the predialysis total subcutaneous dose. In most cases, 50% of the intraperitoneal dose is used for the long dwell daytime exchange, with the remaining 50% equally divided among the nocturnal exchanges.

The 1 year patient survival for diabetic patients on CCPD is reported to be about 75%. The main indications for CCPD in diabetics include young diabetics awaiting cadaveric or living related renal transplantations, and older, blind, and dependent diabetics requiring partner help to perform dialysis technique. Those patients who develop complications due to the increased intra-abdominal pressure, may be given CCPD with a low volume daytime exchange. Another group of patients who benefit from CCPD with a low daytime volume are those who complain of chronic low back pain on CAPD.

Continuous ambulatory peritoneal dialysis (CAPD)

The technique of CAPD is usually modified to accommodate patient handicaps so as to allow them to self-perform dialysis at home. Devices such as the ultraviolet box, splicer, Oreopoulos–Zellerman connector, Y-transfer set with a UV system, and injecta aid, etc., are used successfully to make them independent.

Blood-sugar control in CAPD patients

The aim of the treatment is to achieve a fasting blood sugar 140 mg/dl, and postmeal (breakfast, lunch, and supper) levels below 200 mg/dl at all times and a glycosylated hemoglobin of 9% or below. Different methods of blood-sugar control in CAPD patients are listed in Table 24. Not all patients can be maintained on IP insulin because of the individual patient variations, preferences, and insulin responsiveness. Recent surveys of blood-sugar control during CAPD by the National CAPD Registry in 487

TABLE 24. Different methods of blood-glucose control during CAPD

1. Intraperitoneal insulin
2. Subcutaneous insulin
3. Combination of IP and SC insulin
4. Oral agents
5. Oral agents and insulin (IP or SC)
6. Diet
7. Diet and oral agents

CAPD patients indicated that approximately 47% of the surveyed patients use IP insulin for their blood-sugar control, 30% use subcutaneous insulin, and the rest of the patients either require no insulin or are on subcutaneous insulin and oral hypoglycemic agents.

No single method is suitable for all patients. In general, noninsulin-dependent diabetics may require only diet and/or oral hypoglycemic agents. Whenever they require insulin, the amount needed to control the blood sugar may be very high because of the high prevalence of insulin resistance.

Intraperitoneal insulin

Most of the insulin secreted by the pancreas is transported to the liver via the portal vein and 50% of the portal venous insulin is extracted by the liver before reaching the systemic circulation (Figure 41). This relatively high concentration of insulin in the liver promotes metabolic modulation of absorbed nutrients before they enter the systemic circulation and is likely to be important in the normal glucose homeostasis. Insulin administered into the peritoneal cavity is partly absorbed by diffusion across the visceral peritoneum into the portal venous circulation and partly through the capsule of liver and, thus, simulates the physiological insulin secretion (Figure 41). Intraperitoneally administered insulin also reaches the systemic circulation rather slowly, by the peritoneal cavity lymphatics.

IP administration of regular insulin promotes the control of glycemia throughout the dwell time; IP insulin is absorbed along with the obligatory glucose load from the dialysis solution and insulin absorption continues until the end of the dwell. Peak insulin levels in the serum are observed 30 to 45 minutes after its administration into an empty peritoneal cavity and delayed until 90 to 120 minutes when insulin is added to the dialysis solution. Approximately 50% of the insulin instilled into the peritoneal cavity is absorbed after an 8 hour dwell time.

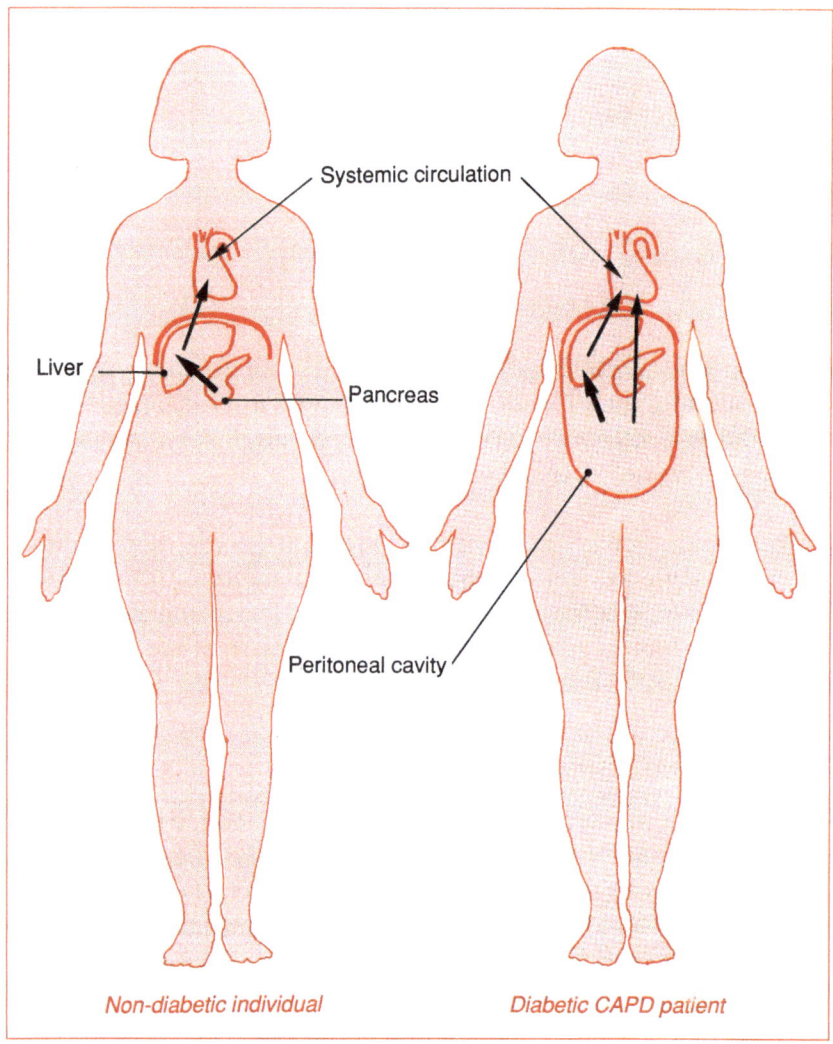

Non-diabetic individual   Diabetic CAPD patient

Figure 41: Insulin kinetics in a nondiabetic normal individual and in a SAPD patient receiving intra-peritoneal (IP) insulin.

The guidelines for IP insulin administration are given in Table 25. IP insulin therapy reduces the meal-related hyperglycemia and daily glucose fluctuations. If care is not exercised, severe fatal hypoglycemia can be encountered with IP insulin administration especially during the night.

IP insulin requirements during episodes of peritonitis are either increased or decreased, depending upon the relative importance of increased insulin absorption and reduced carbohydrate intake due to anorexia versus increased glucose absorption and the infection-related catabolic state.

There are physiological similarities between the uptake of endogenous insulin in normal persons and in CAPD patients taking IP insulin.

Short-term and long-term outcomes

The 3-year cumulative survival rate on CAPD is significantly better than that achieved by intermittent peritoneal dialysis because of the better solute clearances during CAPD and better control of blood pressure. However, the actuarial survival and technique success rates for diabetics are lower than in nondiabetics of comparable age on CAPD. The reported 3-year survival rates for diabetics range from 40 to 60% depending on the age of the patients. The outcome of treatment in noninsulin-dependent

TABLE 25. Guidelines for blood-sugar control with IP insulin administration in a standard CAPD patient

1. The dialysis exchanges are performed during the day to coincide with the major meals, i.e., breakfast, lunch, and supper. The fourth exchange is made at around 2300 hours, at which time a small snack may be taken.
2. The patient is advised to consume a diet providing 20–25 kcal/kg body weight/day and containing protein of 1.2 to 1.5 g/kg BW.
3. During the initial control, blood sugar by finger prick method is estimated 4 times a day, pre-exchange.
4. After cleaning the blood port of the dialysis solution bag with a sterilizing solution, and using a syringe with a long needle, regular insulin is added to each dialysis solution bag. The time of insulin injection into the bag, prior to solution infusion should be standardized. The bag is inverted 2 or 3 times to aid mixing.
5. At the initiation of CAPD, 150% of the pre CAPD daily subcutaneous insulin dose can be safely divided among all 4 exchanges, with a reduced insulin dose added to the overnight dwell to avoid nocturnal hypoglycemia.
6. Review of pre-exchange blood-glucose results allows stepwise changes in insulin added to each cycle until desired blood-glucose control is achieved.
7. Increments in insulin are required for each additional hypertonic dialysis cycle incorporated into the daily routine. Increments differ among patients. An individual patient's requirement should be determined at the time of training.
10. Patients are trained to check their blood-sugar levels with the finger-prick method. This method, which gives quick results, and correlates well with the venous blood sugar levels, helps to detect unexpected fluctuations in blood sugar. The finger-prick test is performed 5 to 10 minutes before each bag exchange and, whenever necessary, the dose of insulin added in the next bag is adjusted according to the guidelines taught to individual patient at the time of training.

diabetes is poorer compared to insulin-dependent diabetes because, as a group, they are older, usually have severe ischemic heart disease, and generally have other associated medical problems.

During the early years of CAPD, it was feared that long-term CAPD in diabetics might not be feasible because of diffuse microvascular disease. Lower solute and water clearances were predicted for diabetics compared to nondiabetics. In addition, concern, due to membrane injury from high rates of peritonitis, led most to predict a short life for the peritoneal membrane and a high dropout from the therapy after a short period was expected. Contrary to the earlier expectations, however, a recent experience in a large group of CAPD patients reported similar peritoneal transport characteristics (based on the peritoneal equilibration studies) for both diabetics and nondiabetics. Although experiences with long-term survival of diabetics on CAPD are very limited, diabetic patients who have been successfully managed on CAPD for longer than 5 years are being reported. Characteristically, the patients who survive long tend to be free from associated cardiac disease, and are nonsmokers. The actuarial survival was 44% at 5 years (26 patients at risk) in one of the series. The NIH CAPD registry survey reported that, of the 7161 CAPD patients surveyed, 19% were on treatment for 3 years or more. Thus, it is becoming apparent that compared to nondiabetic patients, diabetic patients on CAPD tend to have lower survival rates and drop out at a higher rate.

> Peritoneal membrane function as assessed by the serum chemistries and equilibration studies remains stable in diabetic CAPD patients over 5 to 6 years.

Compared to diabetic patients on hemodialysis, the survival on CAPD may not be very much different. However, compared with nondiabetics on any form of dialysis and after kidney transplantation, the outcome of both hemo- and peritoneal dialysis in diabetics is poorer mainly because of the coexistence of other medical problems.

The complications observed in diabetics on CAPD are similar to nondiabetics on CAPD. Complications which are a direct result of increased intra-abdominal pressures, such as dialysate leaks, hernia, hemorrhoids, and a compromised cardiac pulmonary status, occur with the same frequency in diabetics as in nondiabetics.

Transient loss of ultrafiltration during an episode of peritonitis is frequent, but full recovery is expected after a period of peritoneal membrane rest. Irreversible loss of ultrafiltration, as in the nondiabetic, may occur in diabetic CAPD patients mainly as a sequela of severe peritonitis and due to sclerosing peritonitis. Although the exact etiology of sclerosing peritonitis has not been established, its occurrence, once most prevalent in Europe, has been almost eliminated since the replacement of acetate buffer by lactate in the dialysis solution.

Most insulin-dependent diabetics have irreversible retinal lesions before they start dialysis, especially during the terminal phase of renal failure when hypertension tends to be severe. In the great majority, by the time they reach the stage of dialysis, ocular lesions are far too advanced to expect any useful recovery. The common lesions seen at the time of initiating CAPD are background retinopathy, proliferative retinopathy, and vitreous hemorrhage. Retinal detachment may also be seen in some cases. Therefore, better preservation of ocular function depends on the more aggressive approach to blood pressure and glucose control during the predialysis phase. Retinal ischemia may be made worse by the rapid fluctuations in the intravascular volume during an intermittent therapy. CAPD avoids many of the problems inherent in the intermittent forms of dialysis. To preserve a useful visual function, some patients may require vitrectomy. Stabilization or even improvement of ocular function in diabetic patients maintained on CAPD has been reported by several centers.

Morbidity and mortality due to atherosclerotic heart disease and microangiopathy remain the main causes of death among diabetics undergoing peritoneal dialysis. Small-vessel disease leading to ischemic gangrene of the extremities is a common complication of type I diabetes. Short-term experiences with CAPD in diabetics do not suggest that ischemic complications occur any more frequently in diabetics than in nondiabetics. In the only long-term experience reported by Zimmermann *et al.*, the incidence of ischemic and/or gangrenous complications was extremely low. The key to preserving adequate circulation to extremities include avoidance of smoking, hypotensive episodes and lipid derangements.

Diabetics on CAPD tend to have increased morbidity and require more frequent hospitalization than nondiabetic patients mainly because of the numerous associated medical problems due to diabetes. For type I and type II diabetics, the rates of hospitalization (33 days per patient year of treatment) appear to be similar. Hospitalization due to causes directly related to CAPD technique are progressively decreasing. The rate of hospitalization for diabetics on CAPD is comparable to diabetics on hemodialysis.

Theoretically, CAPD may be associated with steady glomerular capillary pressure in the remaining functioning glomeruli without any fluctuations to high or low levels. This feature of CAPD may have a protective effect on residual renal function. Several prospective and cross-sectional studies compared endogenous creatinine clearances in diabetic patients on CAPD and hemodialysis. All studies showed a greater decline in the residual function in patients on hemodialysis compared to CAPD patients. Several explanations have been proposed for faster decline in residual renal function in patients on HD:

(1) glomerular ischemia during hypotension,
(2) glomerular capillary hypertension with volume expansion, and
(3) blood membrane interaction with release of nephrotoxic cytokines.

Preserving the residual renal function has clinical implications in the dialysis prescription, and fluid, sodium, and potassium balance during dialysis treatment.

11 PERITONEAL DIALYSIS IN CHILDREN

Continuous ambulatory peritoneal dialysis (CAPD), when introduced in adults in the late seventies, became the preferred chronic dialytic therapy for children, primarily because of its simplicity and some additional social and medical advantages, previously discussed.

Peritoneal physiology

Infants have more than twice the peritoneal surface area per unit weight than adults.

> Although the data are sparse, it is now believed that with appropriate size adjustments, peritoneal membrane permeability for most small solutes are similar in children and adults.

Reduced net ultrafiltration in children probably reflects mainly higher rates of lymphatic absorption per kg body weight. Adjusted glucose absorption rates may be slightly higher because of the relatively greater peritoneal surface area per unit body weight; however, the increased area

TABLE 26. Steps of temporary peritoneal access for small infants

1. An area in the midline one-third of the way below the umbilicus is anesthetized and an incision is made.
2. A 16 gauge angio-catheter is used to enter the abdomen and the needle is removed.
3. A guide wire is placed through the angio-catheter into the abdomen.
4. A Sheldon catheter is placed over the wire and into the abdomen.
5. The catheter is fixed with tape and dialysis is initiated.

would allow more UF at a lower osmotic gradient. The relative increased area might have little effect on transcapillary UF or net UF per unit body weight because of these countering effects.

Peritoneal access

The peritoneal access is obtained by either rigid or silastic Tenckhoff catheters. The steps of obtaining a peritoneal access in infants are given in Table 26. This approach provides a rapid peritoneal access. Peritonitis and outflow obstruction are the two common problems observed with this approach of peritoneal access. It is easy to replace a new catheter through a guide wire in the case of outflow obstruction which is mainly due to omental capture of the catheter.

Tenckhoff catheter insertion is usually done surgically. A purse-string suture is placed around the cuff close to the peritoneum for good seal. Lateral insertion minimizes dialysis solution leak.

> To minimize the problem of omental capture of catheters, some insert the internal segment of the catheter through a window in the omentum. Others perform partial omentectomy.

Acute renal failure

The convenience, simplicity, and relative safety of peritoneal dialysis allow the nephrologist to initiate dialysis in a child with acute renal failure, as soon as it is needed. Absolute contraindications to peritoneal dialysis in children are few, and all are those in whom an intact peritoneal cavity is lacking. Patients with different types of stomas, prune-belly syndrome, polycystic kidneys, recent bowel surgeries, etc., have all received successful peritoneal dialysis at many centers. The mechanics of dialysis are similar to that in adults.

> Newer cyclers, capable of delivering small volumes of solution, have made peritoneal dialysis easy to institute for children.

Similar to adults, peritonitis is the most frequent complication when a rigid catheter is used for access. Metabolic disturbances can easily occur during acute dialysis and, therefore, close monitoring is suggested for all acute dialysis in children.

End-stage renal disease

The choice of peritoneal dialysis over hemodialysis is based on the multiple factors, which are listed in Table 27.

Continuous peritoneal dialysis regimen, such as CAPD or CCPD is preferred over intermittent regimen because of better small solute clearances. The recommended dialysis solution volume per exchange is 2000 ml/m^2. The number of exchanges performed per day vary between 4 and 5. Most of the clinical benefits of CAPD observed in adults have also been seen in children. Because of the parental convenience, CCPD is preferred over CAPD in children.

The major concern of pediatric nephrologists with regards to CAPD in children relates to nutrition and growth. Many young children on CAPD show improved nutritional status compared to predialysis state but are still malnourished, as evidenced by the low serum albumin levels. Protein losses contribute in a significant way to malnutrition. Patients who are force-fed through nutritional supplements or tube feedings, show signs of nutritional gains, such as weight gain, increased muscle mass, and/or skin fold thickness.

Current dietary recommendations for an infant/child on CAPD are to provide an energy intake of at least 100% of the recommended dietary allowances (RDA) for children of the same sex and age-height. Total energy intake is augmented by an additional 18–20 kcal/kg/day derived from glucose absorbed from the dialysis solution. The available data are insufficient to determine the minimal protein intake required to achieve positive nitrogen balance in pediatric CAPD patients of different ages. The current recommendations are to ensure a minimum daily protein intake of 2 g/kg for children >2 years of age. Water soluble vitamins are supplemented in every CAPD patient. On CAPD, the majority of children grow at rates >70% of expected, but catch-up growth does not occur.

The use of a recombinant growth hormone suggests that adequate growth can be achieved in these children on CAPD/CCPD.

TABLE 27. Factors that influence the choice of peritoneal dialysis over hemodialysis in infants and children

1. Difficult vascular access in small children
2. Technical difficulties of hemodialysis
3. PD is more easily adapted for home dialysis
4. Distance from the center

Complications observed during CAPD in children are similar to those seen in adults on CAPD. The majority of children on CAPD experience progression of renal osteodystrophy, despite treatment with vitamin D analogues, calcium, and phosphate binders. If a mild degree of hypercalcemia is maintained with calcitriol, improvement in bone disease can be expected. As in adults, calcium-containing phosphate binders are effective in lowering phosphate levels. Aluminum-containing phosphate binders should be avoided.

Peritonitis rates in experienced hands are lower with CCPD than CAPD. However, with the use of Y-transfer sets, these differences are decreasing. The spectrum of peritonitis and its management in children is similar to that in adult CAPD patients.

Survival rates on CAPD/CCPD are lower in children compared to adults. Infants and younger children have higher rates of mortality compared to older children.

The most impressive feature of CAPD in children is the remarkable improvement in the quality of life of patients and their families. Not only does CAPD/CCPD free the patients from the limitations of in-center hemodialysis, but it promotes independence and self-reliance. It also gives families an opportunity to participate in their children's treatment.

LITERATURE FOR FURTHER READING

Recommended Books for further reading:

Peritoneal Dialysis, Nolph KD (ed), Kluwer Academic Publishers, Dordrecht, The Netherlands, 3rd edition, 1989

Advances in Peritoneal Dialysis – Yearly publication of selected papers from the Annual Conference on Peritoneal Dialysis, Peritoneal Dialysis Bulletin, Inc. Toronto Publishers.

Chapters and Articles

Alexander SR. Peritoneal dialysis in children. In: Nolph KD (ed), Peritoneal Dialysis, 3rd ed., Kluwer Academic Publishers, Dordrecht, pp 343-364, 1989.

Amair P, Khanna R, Leibel B, et al. Continuous ambulatory peritoneal dialysis in diabetics with end stage renal disease. N Eng J Med 306:625-630, 1982.

Arfania D, Everett ED, Nolph K, Rubin J. Uncommon causes of peritonitis in patients undergoing peritoneal dialysis. Arch Int Med 141:61-64, 1981.

Ash SR, Johnson H, Hartman J, et al. The column disc peritoneal catheter. A peritoneal access device with improved drainage. ASAIO J 3:109-115, 1980.

Bargman JM, Oreopoulos DG. Complications other than peritonitis or those related to the catheter and the fate of uremic organ dysfunction in patients receiving peritoneal dialysis. In: Nolph KD (ed), Peritoneal Dialysis, 3rd ed., Kluwer Academic Publishers, Dordrecht, pp 289-318, 1989.

Bazzato G, Coli U, Landini S, et al. Xylitol and low dosages of insulin: New perspectives for diabetic uremic patients on CAPD. Perit Dial Bull 2:161-164, 1982.

Benevent D, Peryonnet P, Brignon P. Urokinase infusion for obstructed catheters and peritonitis. Perit Dial Bull 5:77, 1985.

Buoncristiani U, Altieri P, Cairo G, Quintaliani G, Ferrara R, Scanziana L. Suitability of CAPD for long term treatment of uremic diabetics. Perit Dial Bull 7(suppl 2):S11, 1987.

Buoncristiani U, Cozzari M, Quintaliani G, Carobi C. Abatement of exogenous peritonitis using the Perugia CAPD system. Dial Tranplant 12:14-25, 1983.

Courtice FC, Steinbeck AW. The rate of absorption of heparinized plasma and of 0.9% NaCl from the peritoneal cavity of the rabbit and guinea-pig. Austr J Exp Biol Med Sci 28:171, 1950.

Daly BDT, Dasse KA, Haudenschild CC, et al. Percutaneous energy transmission systems: Long-term survival. Trans Am Soc Artif Intern Organs 29:526-530, 1983.

Daugirdas JR, Ing TS, Gandhi VC, Hano JE, Chen WT, Yuan L. Kinetics of peritoneal fluid absorption (from the peritoneal cavity) in patients with chronic renal failure. J Lab Clin Med 95:351, 1980.

Delmez JA, Dougan CS, Gearing BK, et al. The effects of intraperitoneal cacitriol on calcium and parathyroid hormone. Kidney Int 31(3):795-799, 1987.

Diaz-Buxo JA. CCPD is even better than CAPD. Kidney Int 28:S26-28, 1985.

Diaz-Buxo JA, Chandler JT, Farmer CD, Smith DL. Chronic peritoneal dialysis at home – a comparison with hemodialysis. Trans Am Soc Artif Intern Organs 23:191-193, 1977.

Diaz-Buxo JA, Gissinger WT. Single cuff versus double cuff Tenckhoff catheter. Perit Dial Bull 4(suppl 3):S100-S102, 1984.

Diaz-Buxo JA, Kay DA, Holt KL. Safe, simple, inexpensive disconnecting device for CCPD. Kidney Int 27:179, 1985.

Diaz-Buxo JA, Walker PJ, Burgess WP, et al. The influence of peritoneal dialysis on the outcome of transplantation. Int J Artif Organs 9:359-362, 1986.

Flessner MF, Enstermacher JD, Blasberg RG, et al. Peritoneal absorption of macromolecules studes by quantitative autoradiography. Am J Physiol 248:H26-H32, 1985.

Flynn CT. Long-term continuous ambulatory peritoneal dialysis. Proc Eur Dial Transpl Assoc 20:700-704, 1983.

Gokal R, Ellis HA, Ward MK, Kerr DNS. Histological renal bone disease in patients on continuous ambulatory peritoneal dialysis. In: Moncrief J, Popovich R (eds), Proc CAPD Int Symp II, Masson, Pub, Austin, TX, p 249, 1980.

Gotloib L, Nisencorn J, Garmizo AL, Galili N, Servadio C, Sudarsky M. Subcutaneous intraperitoneal prosthesis for maintenance peritoneal dialysis. Lancet i:1318-1319, 1975.

Grefberg N. Clinical aspects of CAPD. Scand J Urol and Nephrology S72:7-38, 1983.

Hau T, Ahrenholz DH, Simmons RL. Secondary bacterial peritonitis: The biologic basis of treatment. In: Current problems in surgery. vol. 16, No. 10. Year Book Medical Publ. Incl, Chicago, 1979.

Heide B, Pierratos A, Khanna R, et al. Nutritional status of patients undergoing continuous ambulatory peritoneal dialysis. Perit Dial Bull 3:138-141, 1983.

Karnovsky MJ. The ultrastructural basis of transcapillary exchanges. In: Biological interfaces: Flows and exchanges. Little Brown, Boston, pp 64-95, 1968.

Katirtzolgou A, Izatt S, Oreopoulos DG. Chronic peritoneal dialysis in diabetics with end stage renal failure. In: Friedman EA, L'Espereance F (eds), Diabetic renal retinal syndrome 2. Grune and Stratton, New York, pp 317-332, 1982.

Keane WF, Everett ED, Fine RN, Golper TA, Vas SI, Peterson PD. CAPD related peritonitis management and antibiotic therapy recommendations: Travenol peritonitis management advisory committee. Perit Dial Bull 7:55-68, 1987.

Khanna R, Izatt S, Burke D, Mathews R, Vas S, Oreopoulos DG. Experience with the Toronto Western Hospital permanent peritoneal catheter. Perit Dial Bull 4:95-98, 1984.

Khanna R, Oreopoulos DG, Dombros N, et al. Continuous ambulatory peritoneal dialysis after three years: Still a promising treatment. Perit Dial Bull 1:24-34, 1981.

Khanna R, Oreopoulos DG, Vas SI, McCready W, Dombros N. Fungal peritonitis in patients undergoing chronic intermittent or continuous peritoneal dialysis. Proc EDTA 17:291-96, 1980.

Khanna R, Twardowski ZJ. Peritoneal dialysis access. In: Nolph KD (ed), Peritoneal dialysis, 3rd ed., Kluwer Academic Publishers, Dordrecht, pp 319-342, 1989.

Kjellstrand C, Whitley K, Comty C, Shapiro F. Dialysis in patients with diabetes mellitus. Diabetic Nephropathy 2:5-17, 1983.

Lindholm B, Bergstrom J. Nutritional management of patients undergoing peritoneal dialysis. In: Nolph KD (ed), Peritoneal dialysis, 3rd ed., Kluwer Academic Publishers, Dordrecht, pp 230-260, 1989.

Mactier RA, Khanna R, Moore H, Russ J, Nolph KD, Groshong T. Kinetics of peritoneal dialysis in children: Role of lymphatics. Kidney Int 34:82, 1988.

Mactier R, Khanna R, Twardowski Z, Nolph K. Role of peritoneal cavity lymphatic absorption in peritoneal dialysis. Kidney Int 32: 1987.

Maiorca R, Cancarini GC, Broccoli R, et al. Prospective controlled trial of a Y-connector and disinfectant to prevent peritonitis in continuous ambulatory peritoneal dialysis. Lancet ii:642-644, 1983.

Matthys E, Dolkart R, Lameire N. Extended use of a glycerol-containing dialysate in diabetic CAPD patients. Perit Dial Bull 7:10-19, 1987.

Mistry CD, Mallick NP, Gokal R. The use of large molecular weight glucose polyper (MW 20.000) as an osmotic agent in continuous ambulatory peritoneal dialysis. In: Khanna R, Nolph KD, Prowant B, Twardowski Z, Oreopoulos DG (eds), Advances in continuous ambulatory peritoneal dialysis, Perit Dial Bull, Inc., Toronto, 6:7-11, 1986.

Moncrief JW, Popvich RP, Nolph KD. Additional experience with continuous ambulatory peritoneal dialysis (CAPD). Trans Am Soc Artif Intern Organs 24:4760-483, 1978.

Nissenson AR, Gentile DE, Soderblom RE, Brax C. Long-term outcome of continuous ambulatory peritoneal dialysis. Trans Am Soc Artif Intern Organs 32(1):560-563, 1986.

Nolph KD. Peritoneal dialysis. In: Drukker W, Parsons FM, Maher JF (eds), Replacement of renal function by dialysis. Martinus Nijhoff Medical Division, The Hague, pp 277-321, 1978.

Nolph KD, Hano JE, Teschan PE. Peritoneal sodium transport during hypertonic peritoneal dialysis: Physiologic mechanisms and clinical implications. Ann Intern Med 70:931-941, 1969.

Nolph KD, Mactier RA, Khanna R, Twardowski ZJ, Moore H, McGary T. The kinetics of ultrafiltration during peritoneal dialysis: The role of lymphatics. Kidney Int 32:219, 1987.

Nolph KD, Miller FN, Rubin J, Popovich R. New directions in peritoneal dialysis concepts and applications. Kidney Int 18 (suppl 10):S111, 1980.

Oren A, Wu G, Anderson G, Marliss E, et al. Effective use of amino-acid dialysate over four weeks in CAPD patients. Am Soc Art Int Organs 29:604-610, 1983.

Oreopoulos DG, Izatt S, Zellerman G, Karanicolas S, Mathews RE. A prospective study of the effectiveness of three permanent peritoneal catheters. Proc Clin Dial Transplant Forum 6:96-100, 1976.

Oreopoulos DG, Khanna R, McCready W, Katirtzoglou A, Vas S. Continuous ambulatory peritoneal dialysis in Canada. Dial Transpl 9:224-226, 1980.

Palmer RA, Maybee TK, Henry EW, Eden J. Peritoneal dialysis in acute and chronic renal failure. Can Med Assoc J 88:920-927, 1963.

Price JDE, Moriarty MV. Continuous ambulatory peritoneal dialysis: Selection criteria – Failures and causes – Deaths – Diabetes mellitus. In: Legrain M (ed), Continuous ambulatory peritoneal dialysis, Excerpta Medica, Amsterdam, pp 113-119, 1980.

Rottembourg J. Peritoneal dialysis in diabetics. In: Nolph KD (ed), Peritoneal dialysis, 3rd ed., Kluwer Academic Publishers, Dordrecht, pp 365-379, 1989.

Rottembourg J, El Shahat Y, Agrafiotis A, et al. Continuous ambulatory peritoneal dialysis in insulin dependent diabetics: A 40 month experience. Kidney Int 23:40-45, 1983.

Rottembourg J, Issad B, Poignet JL, et al. Residual renal function and control of blood glucose levels in insulin-dependent diabetic patients treated by CAPD. In: Keen H, Legrain M (eds), Prevention and treatment of diabetic nephropathy. MTP Press, Lancaster, pp 339-352, 1983.

Rubin J. Comments on dialysis solution, antibiotic transport, poisonings, and novel uses of peritoneal dialysis. In: Nolph KD (ed), Peritoneal dialysis, 3rd ed., Kluwer Academic Publishers, Dordrecht, pp 199-229, 1989.

Rubin J, Oreopoulos DG, Lio TT, Mathews R, deVeber GA. Management of peritonitis and bowel perforation during chronic peritoneal dialysis. Nephron 16:220-225, 1976.

Schade DS, Eaton RP, Spencer W. The advantages of peritoneal route of insulin delivery. In: Irsigler K, Kunz KN, Owen DR, Regal H (eds), New approaches to insulin therapy, MTP Press, Lancaster, pp 31-39, 1981.

Slingeneyer A, Canaud B, Mion C. Permanent loss of ultrafiltration capacity of the peritoneum in long-term peritoneal dialysis: An epidemiological study. Nephron 33:133, 1983.

Spencer PC, Farrell PC. Applications of kinetic monitoring in CAPD. In: Weimar W, Fieren MWJA, Diderich PPNN (eds). Continuous ambulatory peritoneal dialysis, Proceedings of the Fourth Benelux Symposium, Rotterdam, November 24, op de Hoek CT. pp 9-23, 1984.

Tenckhoff H. Peritoneal dialysis today: A new look. Nephron 12:420-436, 1974.

Tenckhoff H, Schechter H. A bacteriologically safe peritoneal access device. Trans Am Soc Artif Intern Organs 14:181-186, 1968.

Tenckhoff H, Schilipeter G, Boen ST. One year experience with home peritoneal dialysis. Trans Am Soc Artif Intern Organs 11:11-14, 1965.

Tenckhoff H, Ward G, Boen ST. The influence of dialysate volume and flow rate on peritoneal clearance. Proc Eur Dial Transpl Assoc 2:113-117, 1965.

Twardowski ZJ, Khanna R, Nolph KD. Osmotic agents and ultrafiltration in peritoneal dialysis. Nephron 42:93, 1986.

Twardowski ZJ, Khanna R, Nolph KD. Peritoneal dialysis modifications to avoid CAPD dropouts. In: Khanna R et al. (eds), Advances in continuous ambulatory peritoneal dialysis. Proceedings of the Seventh Annual CAPD Conference, Kansas City, Missouri, February 1987. Peritoneal Dialysis Bulletin, Incl, Toronto. pp 171-178, 1987.

Twardowski ZJ, Khanna R, Nolph KD, et al. Intraabdominal pressure during natural activities in patients treated with continuous ambulatory peritoneal dialysis. Nephron 44:129-135, 1986.

Twardowski ZJ, Nichols WK, Khanna R, Nolph KD. Swan neck peritoneal dialysis catheters: Design, features, sterilizing, insertion and break-in. Instruction manual published by: Accurate Surgical Instruments Corp., 588-590 Richmond St. W., Toronto, Ontario, Canada M5V 1Y9, 1986.

Twardowski ZJ, Nolph KD, Khanna R, Gluck Z, Prowant BF, Ryan LP. Daily clearances with continuous ambulatory peritoneal dialysis and nightly peritoneal dialysis. Trans Am Soc Artif Intern Organs 32: 575-580, 1986.

Twardowski ZJ, Nolph KD, Khanna R, Prowant BF, Ryan LP, Nichols WK. The need for a 'swan neck' permanently bent, arcuate peritoneal dialysis catheter. Perit Dial Bull 5:219-223.

Vas SI. Indications for removal of peritoneal catheter. Perit Dial Bull 1:145-146, 1981.

Vas SI. Microbiologic aspects of chronic ambulatory peritoneal dialysis. Kidney Int 23:83-92, 1983.

Vas SI, Low DE, Layne S, Khanna R, Dombros N. Microbiological diagnostic approach to peritonitis in CAPD patients (1981). In: Atkins RC et al. (eds), Peritoneal Dialysis. Churchill Livingstone, Edinburgh, pp 269-271, 1981.

Wayland H, Silberberg A. Blood to lymph transport. Microvasc Res 15:367, 1978.

Wood C, Thomson NM, Scott DF, et al. Results of renal transplantation in patients on CAPD. Perit Dial Bull 4:S72, 1984.

Zimmerman SW, Johnson CA, O'Brien M. Survival of diabetic patients on CAPD for over five years. Perit Dial Bull 7:26-29, 1987.

INDEX

acinetobacter 76, 77
acquired cystic disease of the kidney 96
acute renal failure 62
adequacy 1
adhesions 87
advantage of APD 67
aluminum toxicity 94
amino acids 101
aminoglycosides 84
anabolic state 89
antibiotic prophylaxis 88
antifungal agents 85
APD 64
   therapy 67
aplastic bone disease 93
assist devices 51
automated peritoneal dialysis (ADP) 64

basement membranes 5, 7
bedside insertion of a catheter 19
bleeding 56
blood-sugar control 105
   in CAPD patients 102
   on APD 68
break-in period 31

candida 78
CAPD 36-39
   indications 44
carbon dioxide 6
catheter blockage 56
catheter removal 33
catheters
   Swan Neck Missouri (SNM) 22
   Tenckhoff 20, 21, 57

   Toronto Western (THW) 20, 22
caval circulation 7
CCPD 36-38
   indications 44
CCPD I 39
CCPD II 41
cells 8
cephalosporins 84
children 109, 111
cilium 4
CIPD 36
clinical indices of adequate peritoneal
      dialysis 69
colloids 8
combined creatinine clearance 71
complications 56, 96
   of acute peritoneal dialysis 61
connective tissue 4
constipation 30
contractility 8
convection 9
convective flow 10
costal pain 56
coughing 22
culture-negative (aseptic) peritonitis 78
cycler machines 64
cyclers 53, 66

DAPD 35, 36
desmosomes 5
diabetic ESRD patients 99
diagnosis of peritonitis 78
dialysis 1
   solution 1, 45
   solution leakage 33, 60

diffusion 9
    rate 10

early treatment 83
electrolyte sieving 12
endocrine function 95
eosinophilic peritonitis 78
epigastric artery 7
equilibrium rates
    high 15, 16
    high average 15, 16
    low 15, 16
    low average 15, 16
erythropoietin 92
exit site 29
    care 33
    infection 88
experiences with APD 67
external contamination 76

follicle-stimulating hormone 95

gelatin 101
GFR 100
glycerol 101
Golgi apparatus 5
growth hormone 95
guidewire 24, 59

high dose CADD 39
high dose NIPD 41
high peritoneal transport rates 72
high volume CADD 39
host defenses 8
hypercalcemia 93
hypernatremia 62
hypertension 93
hypotension 78

inclusions 5
indications for APD 66
infants 111
insufficient ultrafiltration 97
intercostal artery 7
intermittent regimens 35
interstitium 5
intraperitoneal fluid 8
intraperitoneal insulin 103
intrathoracic negative pressure 8
IPD 36
    blood-sugar control 101
iPTH 93

Kt/V 73

laboratory indices of adequate peritoneal
    dialysis 69
lactate 45
limitation of APD 68
lipid metabolism 92
lumbar artery 7
luteinizing hormone 95
lymphatic drainage 8

management of peritonitis 83
mass transfer area coefficient 75
mesothelial cells 4
mesothelium 4
metabolic alkalosis 63
microvilli 7
midline insertion 25
mitochondria 5
morbidity 107
mortality 107
mycrobacterium 77

nerve conduction velocities 94
neuropathy 101
NIPD 36, 41
NTPD 41
nuclei 5
nutritional problems 89

organ perforation 60
osmotic agent 13, 101
osmotic ultrafiltration 10
osteitis fibrosa cystica 93
oxygen 6

pain 56
paramedian incision 25
parietal peritoneum 4, 7
PCR 74
peak intraperitoneal volume 14
peak ultrafiltration 18
penicillins 84
pericarditis 94
peritoneal cavity 4
peritoneal clearance 70
peritoneal equilibration rates 15
peritoneal equilibration test 18
peritoneal membrane 1
    function 106
    sclerosis 88
peritoneoscopic technique 22
peritonitis 76
    during APD 86
    intermittent therapy 76
phosphatidylcholine 4
pinocytosis 13

plasma amino acid levels 90
polyglucose 101
poor drainage 60
portal circulation 7
post-operative care 30
prescription 60
pressure-related complications 96
proportioning units 53
protein 8
protein catabolic rate (PCR) 74
proteoglycan filaments 6
protuberances 7
Pseudomonas sp 76
pseudomonas maltophilia 77

quinolones 85

re-absorption of fluid 14
recurrent peritonitis 86
reduplication 7
reflection coefficient 12
renal osteodystrophy 93
residual renal function 70, 108
retinopathy 101
rigid catheter 54
    insertion 54, 55
rough endoplasmic reticulum 5, 7

sclerosing peritonitis 88
semipermeable 12
shoulder pain 56
sieving coefficient 12
silicone rubber 19
standard dose CAPD 39
standardized peritoneal equilibration test
    15
staphylococcus aureus 77

staphylococcus epidermidis 77
steps of a solution exchange 49, 50
sterile connection device 51
stomata 8
straining 22
streptococcus viridans 77
subcutaneous tunnel 27
superior mesenteric artery 7
surgical technique 25

T_3 95
T_4 95
Tenckhoff catheter 20, 21, 57
testosterone 95
TPD 36
transcapillary ultrafiltration 13, 14
transdiaphragmatic dialysis solution leak
    97
transfer sets 46
trauma 32
TSH 95

ultrafiltration 13, 14
ultraviolet light devices 51
urea kinetics 73
uremic peritoneum 6

vancomycin 85
vascular problems 95
visceral peritoneum 4
vomiting 22

xylitol 101

Y-set procedure 50, 53
Yeast 77